LIZ EARLE'S

A·C·E
PLAN

WEIGHT-LOSS
FOR LIFE

LIZ EARLE

B⊕XTREE

For Paddy

Those who cross the sea change the sky, not their spirits

First published in Great Britain in 1994 by Boxtree Limited,
Broadwall House, 21 Broadwall, London SE1 9PL

Copyright © Liz Earle 1994

10 9 8 7 6 5 4 3 2 1

ISBN: 1 85283 554 0

Cover design: Design 23
Illustrations: Raymond Turvey

Typeset by SX Composing Ltd, Rayleigh, Essex
Printed and bound in Great Britain by Cox & Wyman Ltd.,
Reading, Berkshire

A CIP catalogue entry for this book is available from the British Library

CONTENTS

Acknowledgments

I am indebted to all those who gave so much of their valuable time to help with my research and writing. These include Professor Anthony Diplock, Dr Catherine Rice-Evans, Dr Bruce Ames, Professor Charles Hennekens, Professor Jeffrey Blumberg, Professor William Pryor, Dr Raxit Jariwalla and Dr Derek Shrimpton. Also my thanks to the Vitamin E Information Service, Vitaminfo, Boots Micronutrients Information Service, The Consumer's Association, The Food Commission, Patrick Holford and team at the Institute for Optimum Nutrition and Key Note Publications Ltd. I am also grateful to my ACE researcher Sarah Mobsby and beholden to Annie Bawtree, Val Holmes and Claire Bowles. Many thanks are due to Mike Honey from The Harbour Club for guidance on safe, sensible and effective exercising – and for his personal motivation! I am also grateful to Patrick, Lily, Guy and Laura for their patient recipe-testing.

On a practical note, special thanks are due to my agent Rosemary Sandberg as well as to Michael, David, Wanda, Kate, Nichola, Vicky and all at Boxtree.

Note: Nutritional references taken from McCance and Widdowson, The Composition of Foods, 5th edition, Royal Society of Chemistry, Ministry of Agriculture, Fisheries and Food. Also from the United States Department of Agriculture Data Bank (on-line database), USDA, 1990.

From the author

I have been researching and writing about health and beauty for books and television programmes for more than a decade. It is only now, with the discovery of the ACE vitamins and their role in good health, that I have been able to write the one book that I always wanted to read: Liz Earle's ACE Plan *Weight-Loss For Life*. This book is a medically proven guide to permanent weight-loss. Scores of diet manuals are published every year, so I vowed that I would only ever put pen to paper when I found a regime that actually *worked*. Not just for me, but for everyone, no matter what age, shape, sex or size.

Let's face it, we would all love to have a slim, healthy body. Why else would you be reading this? But *Weight-Loss for Life* is not just about losing weight. It's about gaining a freedom from diets that can't and don't work. Follow this plan and I guarantee you will not only look better, but you will also *feel* better. Slim people have more energy, greater vitality and simply seem able to do more than those weighed down by excess baggage. Being the right weight for our height also increases our life expectancy and protects us against many serious, painful and life-threatening diseases. While I was writing *Liz Earle's ACE Plan*, I discovered that there are many similarities between eating for good health and eating to lose weight. Having always had a tendency to pile on the pounds myself, I was intrigued to find that the same antioxidant ACE vitamins which delay ageing and protect us from heart disease and cancer also have an important role in helping us to lose weight. The ACE vitamins are found in the very foods that help shift excess weight, keep us slim and ensure we stay fit and healthy.

The discovery that the ACE vitamins can help us to achieve a dramatic, permanent weight-loss is exciting news for dieters everywhere. Not only will the antioxidant ACE vitamins help to protect every single cell in the body against the ravages of disease, they will also build a strong, healthy and above all, *slim* physique. Since following the ACE eating guidelines in this book, I have lost over a stone in weight without even trying and have gained a new-found energy and zest for life which was previously missing. For me, and millions of others like me, this new way of eating will become not only a matter of permanent weight-loss, but also of long-term health gain. Good luck with your ACE eating. Remember that you have nothing to lose but your weight.

Liz Earle, 1994

Introduction

The Art of Healthy Slimming

This is the last diet book you will ever need to buy.

The principles of ACE eating not only guarantee that you will lose weight easily, but also ensure you gain better health, renewed energy and improved vitality. *Weight-Loss for Life* is not a fad diet. It is an effective, permanent guide to 'vitality eating'.

The principles of *Weight-Loss for Life* are based on the same sound medical science that has made *Liz Earle's ACE Plan* such a success. In addition to the important diet principles of low-fat, high-fibre foods, this eating programme highlights the importance of the antioxidant ACE super-slimming foods. These are the most important group of foods for giving the body an extra weight-loss boost. The ACE super-slimming foods are packed with energy-giving vitamin A (in the form of beta-carotene), vitamin C and vitamin E. These three nutrients are referred to throughout this book as the ACE vitamins. Switching on to these will make a real difference to the speed at which you lose weight.

While lasting weight-loss is important, lifelong health gain is also a top priority. This book offers you the unique chance to combine the two and get slim while gaining energy from the ACE super-slimming menus. Unlike other fad diets based on pseudo-science and temporary results, this weight-loss guide is all about successful, healthful slimming. It does not offer the false promise of 'get thin quick'. The weight-reduction you will experience will be steady and, above all else, totally permanent. Realistic, achievable goals are set at the end of this chapter and you will be encouraged to make gradual changes to your eating habits, while still eating most of the foods you enjoy. With the help of this book, you will find it surprisingly easy to lose those extra pounds and prevent them from ever returning.

ACE Weight-Loss Charter

The Ace Plan *Weight-Loss for Life* programme makes you the following promises:
- You will lose as much weight as is realistically possible
- You will develop a healthier view of food
- You will boost your health, vitality and energy levels
- You will never need to fad-diet again
- You will burn your food as fuel instead of storing it as excess fat
- You will eat more vitamin-rich foods and protect your health

1
NOT JUST ANOTHER DIET BOOK

Sixty per cent of all women regard themselves as overweight

The last few years have seen more books about diets and regimes to lose weight than on any other subject. So why the need for yet another guide? Well, if any of these books, tapes, videos or charts actually *worked* we'd all have reached our target weight years ago. As it is, far too many of us are grossly overweight. According to the Government *Health of the Nation* Green Paper published in 1991, 45 percent of British males and 36 percent of females are overweight (120 percent or more than optimum weight for frame size). In addition, a 1992 Gallup Poll showed that 59 percent of men and 60 percent of women think of themselves as being overweight. Recognizing this as a serious health problem, the government aims to reduce the number of obese people by at least a quarter for men and a third for women by the year 2005. How does it intend to achieve this? Basically, by encouraging us all to eat less fat.

The government aims to reduce the amount of fat eaten by 12 percent to no more than 35 percent of our total energy intake (we currently get around 42 percent of all our energy from fat in foods). However, it is not enough simply to reduce the fat in our diet. Although this is very important, it is also essential that we increase the amounts of antioxidant ACE vitamins that we eat and this is one of the main aims of this book.

The ACE vitamins have a very special role to play in protecting our health and we shall look more closely at how and why they work in the following chapters. In essence, eating more of the antioxidant ACE vitamins improves our health and cuts our risk of obesity and heart disease. In France, where the daily fat intake is only marginally lower than in Britain, the overall rate of deaths from heart disease is less than a third of ours in the UK: 112 per 100,000 people, per year, compared to 367 per 100,000 in Britain. The best explanation for this extraordinary difference is the ACE vitamins. These are found in colourful fruits and vegetables, cooking oils and nuts. The French eat, on average, 331g of fruit and vegetables a day, against just 187g in Britain. This means they automatically eat a far higher amount of the protective ACE vitamins than we do. By boosting our levels of the ACE vitamins, we can preserve not only our slim figures, but our arteries as well.

Diets can damage your wealth

While the cream, lard and beef suet industries are in for leaner times in the future, the slimming business is booming. In 1992, we spent more than £1.5 *billion* on slimming foods and products. Profits for the food industry are enormous and huge amounts of money are also spent encouraging us to buy 'slimming' aids. For example, Slim Fast meal replacements are backed by a £4 million promotional campaign, St Ivel spend over £2 million a year advertising Shape Yoghurt and even Batchelors Slim-a-Soup enjoys more than a million pounds' worth of advertising each year. But liquid 'diet' drinks, meal replacement bars and small sachets of dehydrated granules are not a natural, vital way of eating. Although highly profitable, they do not teach us the simple eating habits that will result in a visible weight-loss for life.

The bald truth is that 95 percent of us who follow a commercial dieting regime put the weight back on, and more, when we stop. We are far more likely to lose ££s than pounds and there is slim evidence that any of the meal replacements and very low calorie regimes work in the long run. Some slimming foods are a calculated con.

A 1993 survey conducted by the Coronary Prevention Group revealed that many convenience foods labelled 'healthy' or 'low calorie' were not only high in fat but also failed the guidelines for salt, fibre and carbohydrate content drawn up by the Department of Health and the World Health Authority (WHO). Meal replacements, such as cereal bars and biscuits have also come under fire. A survey published in the Food Commission's *Food Magazine* discovered that these may be 'no healthier than a chocolate biscuit or a milk shake.' The article examined 12 products including Slim Fast, Crunch 'n' Slim, Slender Plan, Limmits and Body Plan. The magazine article, entitled *The Slimming Scandal* criticized these meal replacements on the grounds of poor nutrition, for recommending too rapid a weight-loss, not encouraging healthy eating habits and for being far too expensive in relation to their content. The products also failed the standards set out in the draft EC Directive on foods regarding calorie, fat and protein content. This is bad news for British dieters.

Clearly we need better information when it comes to healthy food choices. Unfortunately the Health Education Authority's yearly nutrition budget of under £1 million is dwarfed by the £600 million or more the food industry spends each year on advertising. Manufactured foods are, pound for pound, less nutritious and tend to be more fattening than their raw ingredients. They are too often high in sugar, fat, salt and too low in fibre. For example, a large portion of McDonalds Chicken McNuggets and chips has over 75g of fat, yet only 4g of fibre. One of the aims of this book is to give you the information to make the informed food choices that will lead to your own permanent weight-loss. It also sets out the unbiased, unequivocal facts of successful slimming. *Weight-Loss for Life* gives you the truth, the whole truth and nothing but the truth.

Diets can damage your health

The danger of dieting is in the fast and furious approach. It is a biological fact of life that the more quickly you lose weight, the faster you will put it back on. Slow, sustained weight-loss is the *only* way to reduce body fat and not lose essential lean muscle tissue. For a diet to be truly effective, any weight-loss must be slow in order to be sustained. Weight-loss must also be based on the newly recognized principles of ACE eating and should be combined with a regular exercise regime. This book is not a 'quick fix'. However, it does offer everyone, regardless of their age, the very real chance to achieve significant, long-term weight-loss for a lifetime.

This book is about weight-loss, not starvation. There is no point in following a regime which involves food deprivation, as this will leave you feeling tired, listless and permanently hungry. Instead, you will have the most accurate and up-to-date information on what should be eaten to encourage weight-loss and health-gain. If you follow the guidelines in this book you will never feel hungry, your energy levels will be high and you will enjoy greater protection from disease and premature ageing. Believe me – it cannot fail.

Why most diets don't work

According to the government's 1992 *Dietary and Nutritional Survey of British Adults*, 12 percent of all women and 4 percent of all men are following a rigid dieting regime at any one time. The average length of these diets is six and a half weeks for women and ten weeks for men. So why aren't all these diets working? The plain, unpalatable truth is that short-term, fad diets simply don't lead to long-term weight-loss. In fact, they are quite likely to cause more harm than good. This is because short-term dieting triggers the damaging yo-yo effect. For example, if you start a fad diet that only allows you to eat a few hundred calories a day, the body believes it is at risk of starvation and quickly responds by conserving energy. This leads to a lowering of our basic metabolic rate, which controls how quickly we burn our food as fuel.

The problem with lowering our metabolism is that the body adapts and learns to survive on fewer calories. Scientists have now recognized that once the metabolism has been lowered by frugal eating, it is hard to boost it back to its previous level when you stop the diet. During a period of intense food restriction, you might only be eating around 1000 calories a day, so the body becomes adept at functioning on this low calorific intake. This means that when you return to your previous calorie intake of around 2000 calories a day, the body stores the extra calories in the form of fat. Not only will your lost weight quickly return, but you are also likely to end up feeling constantly hungry and pile on the pounds more easily than before. This yo-yo rebound at the end of a period of dieting is one of the key reasons why so many diets don't work in the long-term. The long-term risk factors of crash dieting followed by weight gain also dangerously increase the risk of heart disease and strokes.

American researchers have found that in addition to messing up our metabolism and damaging our health, being on a strict diet actually encourages fat cells to flourish! This is because when we severely restrict our eating, the body protects itself against possible famine by actually storing more fat. Very low-calorie diets simply increase the efficiency of fat storage, so extreme restrictions on eating boosts unwanted fat cells. While this does not mean that we can lose weight by living on cream cakes and chips, it does show that long-term, successful slimming requires a change in tactics from conventional calorie-counting.

The slimming industry's promotion of unhealthy, fad diets is quite simply morally unacceptable. The relentless promotion of so-called diet products puts many millions of women under intense pressure to conform to the advertiser's pin-thin size 8 models, and to feel inadequate if they cannot attain the 'ideal' shape. This book is different. It recognizes that there is no standard weight or size, just broad guidelines which can help us to lose weight and feel fitter at the same time. There is no doubt that faddy eating habits and society's obsession with the svelte female form must also take some blame for the dramatic rise in serious eating disorders over the last decade. It is therefore important to put any kind of weight-loss regime into perspective. This book is not about achieving the impossible: it does not stress starvation tactics or unhealthy self-denial. The weight-loss achieved by adopting the ACE eating principles will be healthy, happy, long-term and above all, effective.

Low-fat, High vitality

The *Weight-Loss for Life* eating regime is entirely safe for every member of the family to follow. This is because it is based on sound nutritional know-how and well-balanced eating. Whether you would like to lose four pounds or forty pounds, the principles of *Weight-Loss for Life* will ensure that the fat not only falls off, but that it stays off forever. The recipes and eating plan have been devised so that they are easy for anyone to follow. They can be adapted to suit teenagers, working women, business dinners, eating out, entertaining, late-night snackers, invalids and the elderly. What is more, once you have achieved your target weight goal, you simply need to stick to the few golden-rules of ACE eating to ensure that those excess pounds never return.

The principles of the *Weight-Loss for Life* regime are remarkably simple. They are based on the guidelines of eating more foods that are rich in vitamin A (in the form of beta-carotene), vitamin C and vitamin E. The many exciting and life-saving properties of these antioxidant nutrients were first explored in *Liz Earle's ACE Plan*. In Chapter Four on page 55 you will find a review of these extraordinary nutrients together with an update of some of the most recent research into their many unique properties. Eating foods that are full of these ACE vitamins automatically boosts our fibre intake and lowers the levels of saturated fat that clogs our system, and feeds our fat cells.

Of all the foods we should be most aware of, fat is the number one enemy of the lean body. Fat contains the highest number of calories, at 9 kcals per gram, than any other type of food. This compares to protein (4 kcals per gram) and carbohydrate (3.75 kcals per gram). This means that it only takes a few grams of fat to start clocking up the calories. By contrast, we can eat almost three times as much carbohydrate as fat – and still lose weight! This is one reason why you will never feel hungry while following this carbohydrate-rich eating regime. Although calorie counting has its critics because it does not take into account the type of food and how it is used in the body (for example, carbohydrates tend to be used as fuel, whereas fats are quickly stored), many of us are happy with the habit of counting calories. For this reason, all the recipes in this book have been calorie-counted. Personally, I prefer not to have to approach each meal with a calculator before eating, although I will concede that calorie counting is a useful tool for getting to grips with the nutritional value of different foods. Each recipe in this book also usefully lists its fat and fibre content, as this information is fundamental to achieving weight-loss. In addition, each recipe details its ACE vitamin content, a unique and very valuable asset for maintaining good health.

Weight-Loss for Life does not insist that you stick to a specific number of calories each day, although the average adult should aim for an intake of 1500-2000 calories a day, depending on frame size, sex and daily energy expenditure. Bear in mind that when a recipe states that it contains a certain number of 'calories' it actually means kilocalories (a kilocalorie is 1000 calories). So, if a dish has 200 kilocalories it is actually 200,000 calories!

The ACE Plan Pyramid

The best way to plan your daily menus is to divide your meals into the different food groups. The following chart shows just what the average weight-loss menu should look like each day.

- 45 percent complex 'starchy' carbohydrates (e.g. wholemeal bread, pasta and potatoes)
- 15 percent protein (e.g. fish, cheese, lean meat and nuts)
- 15 percent saturated fat (e.g. animal fat such as butter, cream and fatty meat)
- 15 percent unsaturated fat (e.g. vegetable oils, most nuts and avocados)
- 10 percent sugar (including honey, glucose, dextrose and all other sugars)

In addition, your daily weight-loss menu should contain the following:
- 15-20 grams of fibre
- 3-5 grams of salt (sodium)
- Less than 300mg of cholesterol (e.g. meat, egg yolks and cream).

The guidelines for ACE eating and weight-loss are easily illustrated in the form of a food pyramid. This at-a-glance picture gives you an instant idea of how to plan your daily meals. The wide bottom of the ACE eating pyramid is the basis for healthy weight-loss and includes 5–9 portions of complex carbohydrates, such as wholemeal bread or

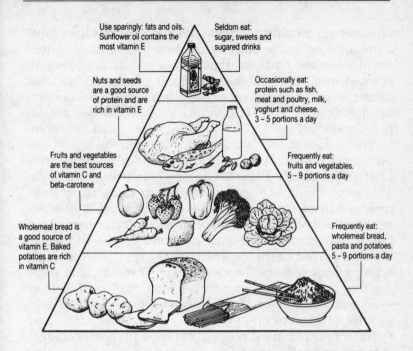

Use sparingly: fats and oils.
Sunflower oil contains the
most vitamin E

Seldom eat:
sugar, sweets and
sugared drinks

Nuts and seeds
are a good source
of protein and are
rich in vitamin E

Occasionally eat:
protein such as fish,
meat and poultry, milk,
yoghurt and cheese.
3 – 5 portions a day

Fruits and vegetables
are the best sources
of vitamin C and
beta-carotene

Frequently eat:
fruits and vegetables.
5 – 9 portions a day

Wholemeal bread is
a good source of
vitamin E. Baked
potatoes are rich
in vitamin C

Frequently eat:
wholemeal bread,
pasta and potatoes.
5 – 9 portions a day

brown rice, each day. The next layer up on the pyramid are the ACE super-slimming foods such as fresh fruits and vegetables. We should aim to eat *at least* 5 portions of these every day. The level above the ACE super-slimming foods consists of a limited amount of protein, such as chicken, fish, meat, eggs and cheese. Protein is often high in fat, so should be eaten sparingly. In this case, between 3–5 servings per day is plenty. At the top of the ACE eating pyramid we find those foods that should be eaten very sparingly. These include fats and oils, sugars, sweets and sugared drinks. These should only be used occasionally as they are all high in calories and often low in ACE vitamins.

How the ACE vitamins work

The ACE vitamins are an exciting discovery for both super-healthy nutrition and effective slimming. The ACE vitamins are all antioxidants, which means that they have a unique role in the body in fighting free radicals. These are dangerous particles that damage cells and lead to many degenerative diseases, including heart disease and cancer. Excessive levels of free radicals also encourage premature ageing. The ACE vitamin foods are the perfect partners for achieving life-long weight-loss and long-term health gain. Not only are these foods naturally low in saturated fat and high in soluble and insoluble fibre, they also contain high levels of energy-enhancing nutrients. This means that ACE eating enables us to be more energetic and to burn our fat supplies faster. The ACE vitamins referred to throughout this book are beta-carotene (which the body turns into vitamin A), vitamin C and vitamin E. There are other nutrients which have a special antioxidant action which will also be mentioned. These include plant extracts and minerals such as selenium. Together they form a powerful team that helps to keep the body young, healthy and full of energy.

The menu-planning recipes and food preparation ideas that follow in the next few chapters focus on choosing ACE vitamin-rich foods, with tips and techniques for preparing, cooking and storing foods to preserve their ACE vitamin levels. All the *Weight-Loss for Life* recipes are not only calorie, fat and fibre counted, they also have a unique ACE vitamin rating. The idea is that you choose from the selection of recipe and menu ideas to plan your ACE-enriched, super-slimming meals. Simply make sure that you eat at least one recipe that highlights a generous level of each of the three ACE nutrients every day.

For example, you could start the day with a breakfast fruit shake (rich in beta-carotene), have an avocado salad with wholemeal pitta bread for lunch (a good source of vitamin E), and finish with watercress soup or a jacket potato for supper (both with plenty of vitamin C). By choosing the recipes in any combination, you can plan the most convenient meals to suit your lifestyle and be safe in the knowledge that you will be boosting your energy-giving ACE vitamins throughout the day. There is also a more structured initial twenty-eight-day eating plan to get you started. Those that like to count calories can also keep tabs on their calorific intake and it is also worth keeping an eye on the amount of fat and fibre in your daily meals to make sure it falls within the guidelines of the ACE Plan Pyramid on page 17.

ACE Weight-Loss Goals

Most of us don't need weight-loss charts to tell us that we need to lose a few pounds, or more. The testing time for our own personal body shape comes when we are in the changing room trying to squeeze into a new size 12 outfit, when buttons on a jacket begin to bulge or when a zip breaks under the strain of our great girth. We all know just by looking in the mirror that we need to lose weight. Unfortunately, research carried out by the National Toxicology Centre in Arkansas, USA, suggests that being slightly *underweight* is actually better for the body. This is because the system has to work less hard to digest food and eliminate toxic and excess materials. Over-eating, bingeing and sheer greed all place a strain on our body.

However, one of the first rules of *Weight-Loss for Life* is to stop weighing yourself more than once a fortnight. It is much more important to lose inches by firming up the body with exercise than it is to lose a few pounds of retained water. Lean muscle weighs more than fat and given the choice, I would far rather be fitter and leaner but weigh *more* than a less fit, plumper person who might actually weigh less than me. It is how you look and feel that is important, not what the scales say. Having said that, it is useful to have some kind of rough guidelines to follow regarding weight. The chart opposite gives you an indication of the optimum weight for your height. However, bear in mind that it is only an indication. A top level athlete will probably weigh more than a couch potato – but I know which one I'd rather look like.

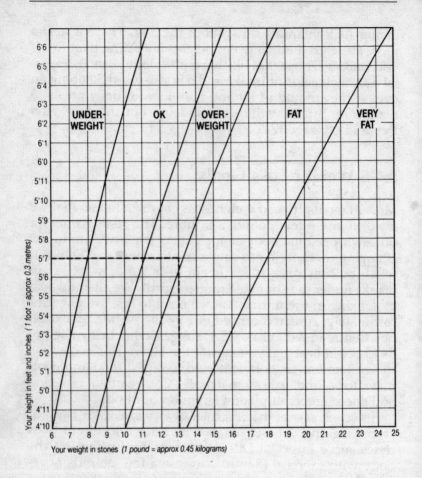

And finally . . .

Before you start your *Weight-Loss for Life* eating regime follow the Dos and Don'ts overleaf.

Dos

- Do believe that *Weight-Loss for Life* will work for you
- Do take one day at a time
- Do forget the 'diet' idea and work towards vitality ACE-eating
- Do look forward to slow, permanent weight-loss
- Do develop a life-long love of fruits and vegetables
- Do ditch the scales
- Do set realistic goals and reward your own efforts with a food-free treat
- Do be patient with your body
- Do make friends with your local greengrocer and become a regular customer
- Do sit down to eat at the table – never eat standing up
- Do only eat when feeling hungry
- Do chew each mouthful more slowly
- Do serve yourself smaller portions
- Do leave a little food on your plate
- Do use smaller plates – a simple trick that fools the brain
- Do have fresh fruit instead of a sugary dessert
- Do clean your teeth after meals to signal the end of eating
- Do remember that muscle weighs more than fat – this means you may even gain weight while exercising but your shape will be leaner
- Do think positive! This regime really does work

Don'ts

- Don't panic! You are not about to be starved or deprived
- Don't skip meals, your body needs a constant energy supply
- Don't feed your fat cells with more fat
- Don't expect results overnight – the more slowly you lose weight, the longer you will keep it off and *Weight-Loss for Life* means forever
- Don't eat late, your body will not be able to burn up the calories before bed
- Don't weigh yourself more than once a fortnight
- Don't eat sweets or chocolate as a pick-me-up
- Don't wear elasticated waistbands – they encourage you to over-eat!
- Don't read or watch TV while eating
- Don't drink with meals. Drink liquids ½ hour before or after eating
- Don't ever have seconds
- Don't visit the supermarket more than once a week – menu planning in advance means you are less likely to buy extra treats
- Don't ever feel guilty about eating – your body needs food, but it needs the *right* kinds of food

2
DIET MAKERS AND BREAKERS

Break bad habits and make friends with good food

Before proceeding with the unique twenty-eight-day starter eating plan that will begin your own personal weight-loss for life, let us first take a closer look at the elements that go into our daily meals. On the one side we have the powerful *diet makers* and on the other we have the destructive *diet breakers*. For successful, permanent weight-loss we need to eat many more of the diet makers and far fewer of the diet breakers. In this chapter we shall examine each of these food allies and foes in turn.

Diet Makers	Diet Breakers
ACE vitamins	Fats
Fibre	Sugars
Exercise	Faddy Eating

- Fats are Fattening
- Carbohydrates are for Fuel

Fats

A low-fat diet is the number one improvement you will make to achieve weight-loss for life and encourage lasting good health. Fats are the cause of excess body fat – not too much starch or carbohydrates. According to the government *Health of the Nation* report, our target for the year 2005 is to have cut our fat intake by at least 12 percent. This means that the average level of fat in the daily diet should fall from about 40 percent to no more than 35 percent. However, in order to achieve lasting weight-loss, our daily fat intake should be between 20 and 30 percent. A minimum fat intake is a fundamental part of healthy eating and is even more of a priority than the other diet issues of sugar, fibre, salt and cholesterol intake. That is not to say that these are not important, just that they are secondary to the fundamental habit of eating much less fat. Remember – fat cells love fat – so don't feed it to them!

In case you are worried that you will miss eating fatty foods, a heartening piece of research was reported in the *American Journal of Clinical Nutrition* in 1993. Studies by nutrition researchers in Philadelphia found that we can all quickly teach ourselves to love a virtually fat-free diet. Over a twelve-week period, researchers found that those on a very low-fat diet reported that they actually *preferred* fat-free eating. After a period of adjustment, almost all the testers decided to continue with their new eating regime because they liked the taste of low-fat foods. Admittedly, the first three months might be tricky for some (so we do need motivation), but in the long-term, this way of eating is actually more enjoyable!

High-Fat Foods	vs	Low-Fat Foods
Cream		Pasta
Butter		Beans and pulses
Cheese		Fish and seafood
Red meat		Breakfast cereals
Egg yolks		Bread
Full fat milk		Fruit and vegetables

Fat-filled Foods

High-fat foods make up a large proportion of our daily diet. 33 percent – cooking fats and vegetable oils make up the lion's share of our fat grammes each day. To reduce this amount, replace hard cooking fats such as lard and suet with a smaller amount of vegetable oil. Grill foods where possible, or dry-fry in a non-stick plan. Where frying is essential, use an oil-spray or remove excess oil from the pan with a paper towel.

26 percent – meat and meat products such as sausages, pâtés and pies are loaded with fat. Always remove visible white fat from meat before grilling or baking. Don't eat sausages, pâté or pies as these are all very high in added fat. Poultry is a lean meat, but always remove high-fat chicken and turkey skin before eating.

22 percent – butter, margarine and 'low-fat' spreads are an obvious source of fat. To cut down on the calories, switch to a reduced fat spread that is whipped with added water.

11 percent – dairy produce and milk are also high in fat. To cut back on the fat-content, use semi-skimmed or skimmed milk instead of full-fat milk. Replace cream with low-fat fromage frais or yogurt and use a reduced-fat cheese.

8 percent – biscuits and cakes account for a considerable number of fat grammes each day. The obvious answer is to cut them out altogether and replace snacking with ACE vitamin-rich fruits, vegetables or fresh fruit juices.

Fat Types

All fats are made up of fatty acids and contain exactly the same number of calories. Fats and oils are equally fattening. However, some fat is far worse for building a healthy body than others. Understanding the vital differences between our everyday fats and oils makes it easy to make the changes that will lead to a leaner, healthier body. Here is the low-down on the different types of fat that we eat.

SATURATES
The reason why a fat becomes 'saturated' has to do with its chemical composition and whether there is room on the fat molecule for hydrogen to bond onto it. Saturated fats are 'fully saturated' and have no room left for extra hydrogen to climb on board. Saturated fats are more easily recognised by being mostly solid at room temperature. Animal fats, such as butter, cheese, lard, dripping, suet and the white fat on meat (including chicken skin) are all very high in saturates. Tropical vegetable oils, such as palm kernel, palm and coconut oils are also high in saturated fats (watch out for these on the ingredient labels of biscuits, cakes and peanut butter).

Conclusion: Saturated fat is the most damaging to our health and has been clearly linked to many forms of cancer and heart disease.

POLYUNSATURATES
The polyunsaturates are 'very-unsaturated' which means that there is plenty of room on their molecule for extra hydrogen bonds. Polyunsaturates are usually found in the form of vegetable oils. The richest source of polyunsaturates are sunflower oil, safflower oil, corn oil and soya oil. These types of fats are thought to be less damaging to our health and they do not clog the arteries in the same way that saturated fats do. However, polyunsaturates are easily broken down by cooking and can turn into potentially dangerous peroxides, which may cause other health problems.

Recent government guidelines not only recommend that we should cut back on overall fat intake, but also suggest that a diet high in polyunsaturates may not be all that good for us. The government committee's report suggests that no more than 10 percent of our daily calories should come from polyunsaturates. This does not sound very much, and it is possible to exceed this if you use a sunflower spread on four slices of bread a day and also use polyunsaturated oils for frying and salad dressings. Eating plenty of vitamin E at the same time as using polyunsaturated oils is essential for good health as the vitamin E protects against the damage caused by free radicals and peroxides.

Conclusion: Small amounts of polyunsaturates are useful in the diet, but should be eaten sparingly. The more polyunsaturates we eat, the more vitamin E we need.

MONOUNSATURATES

The monounsaturate molecule has room for just one hydrogen atom to bond on to it. These fats are probably the healthiest of all as they do not clog the arteries in the same way that saturates can. They are also more stable during frying than the polyunsaturates, so are the best for cooking with. Monounsaturates are mostly liquid at room temperature, but may solidify if stored in the fridge (olive oil is a good example of this). Several vegetable oils are high in monounsaturates including olive, rapeseed, groundnut (peanut), hazelnut, sesame and some blended vegetable oils.

Conclusion: Probably the best of all the fats, mono-unsaturates can be found in many healthy foods such as avocado, oats, nuts and seeds. One of the best all-rounders for cooking is cold-pressed olive oil, which also has a healthy amount of vitamin E.

TRANS FATS

These have been the subject of much of the recent research into healthy eating. Trans fatty acids are naturally present in small amounts in meat and dairy produce. They are also artificially created by the process of hydrogenation. This is when a liquid vegetable oil is hardened by an industrial process using nitrogen and turned into a semi-solid fat. A simple example of this is when sunflower oil is hydro-genated and turned into a sunflower margarine. Unfortu-nately, this common procedure has the side-effect of creat-ing a large number of trans fatty acids. These behave in a similar way to saturated fat and have also been linked to cancer and heart disease. The trans fatty acid content of some margarines is as high as 35 percent, but the manufacturers are not required to state this on the label. This means that those sunflower spreads that fill the chilled cabinets in supermarkets are not quite as healthy as their advertising would have us believe. Fortunately, some un-hydrogenated spreads made with non-hardened oils can be found in health shops. Alternatively, choose the softest type of spread you can find, as this generally contains fewer hardened or hydrogenated oils.

Conclusion: The artificial trans fatty acids from hydrogenated fats crop up in countless other products, including most biscuits, breads and cakes. They are best avoided, so check the label before buying any processed foods.

The recipes and menu suggestions that you will find later on do not include any hydrogenated fats and suggest the use of natural monounsaturates, such as olive oil. However, bear in mind that all vegetable oils are 100 percent pure fat, so no matter which you choose, they will provide you with around 900 calories per 100g. This equals 100 calories per tablespoon. Most solid cooking fats and oils are also 100 percent fat. Fat may be 'hidden' on the label in various guises. The following are all types of fat which you should watch out for:

- partially hydrogenated oils
- vegetable oils
- palm oil
- shortening
- lard
- animal fat
- butter
- cream

Slimmers should use all fats with caution and choose soft low-fat and diet spreads which are whipped with water and contain around 80 percent fat, so have slightly fewer calories. Unhydrogenated diet spreads are hard to find but can be tracked down in the better health food shops.

Fat Substitutes

Instead of encouraging us to eat less fat, the food industry has invested millions of pounds in developing fat-free fats. At first glance these synthetic inventions sound too good to be true – at last we can have fatty foods without the calories. So what's the catch? There are two main problems with these new fat substitutes. Firstly, we do not know what the long-term consequences are of feeding our bodies with unnatural chemical compounds. We are only just beginning to learn of the consequence of hydrogenation and the use of fat within the body is a complex subject. Secondly, artificial fats do nothing to retrain our appetites and encourage vitality eating.

One example of the fat substitutes is Olestra, a non-calorific fat developed by Procter and Gamble for use in a wide range of foods. It is made from a type of sucrose polyester produced by chemically linking several fatty acid molecules to a molecule of sucrose (refined sugar). As sucrose polyester is not a natural substance it is not recognized by the body (we do not have the digestive enzymes needed to digest or absorb it). This means that Olestra and other similar hi-tech inventions are not digested or absorbed, so they provide no calories. Despite extensive laboratory testing, the American consumer watchdog Center for Science in the Public Interest has found that Olestra caused cancer, liver damage and other disorders in animal tests. This organization also concluded that the manufacturer's safety data are currently inadequate and we should caution against the use of synthetic non-fats.

Conclusion: Unfortunately, slimming innovations that sound too good to be true are most often exactly that. Fat-free fats need extensive, long-term testing before they can be considered anything like safe for us and our children to eat. They also ignore the basic health message that the only way permanently to lose weight, gain energy and a zest for life is to eat fewer refined foods and more ACE vitamin-rich fruits, vegetables and whole grains.

Count Your Fat-grams

A healthy diet should contain no more than 35 percent fat, but a weight-loss diet should contain between 20 and 25 percent fat. This level will result in long-term weight-loss as well as dramatically reducing our risk of cancer and heart disease. One of the easiest ways to monitor the amount of fat we eat each day is to keep track of our fat-grams. This method of weight-watching is especially popular in America, where it has largely replaced calorie-counting. In the United States, most foods and many restaurant menus now list their fat-gram content.

The average healthy diet consists of around 80 grams of fat a day, but this should be reduced to 20 to 40 grams of fat a day for dieters. Learning the fat-gram content of foods is actually more effective than counting calories, as it highlights the most fattening forms of foods. Read the labels and look out for fat grams. You can also work out the fat content of foods where it is not shown by multiplying the number of grams of fat in a portion by nine to find out how many calories of fat a serving contains.

- Full-fat milk contains 22g per pint
- Semi-skimmed milk contains 11g per pint
- Skimmed milk contains just 1g fat per pint

By contrast with many of these high-fat foods, see how easy it is to trim fat-grams by switching to lower fat alternatives or by changing the way we cook our food. Simple changes will dramatically alter our food's fat content:

Fried courgette	90% fat	Steamed courgette	0% fat
Breaded & fried cod	62% fat	Grilled cod	7% fat
Baked potato & sour cream	60% fat	Plain baked potato	0% fat
Boiled potatoes & butter	53% fat	Plain boiled potato	0% fat
Chicken roll with mayonnaise	47% fat	Plain chicken roll	16% fat

Fat-gram Finder

Type of food	fat-grams per average-sized portion		
Pork pie	30g		
Samosa	26g		
Streaky bacon, fried	25g	Streaky bacon, grilled	20g
Steak and kidney pie	24g		
Sausages	21g	Fat-reduced sausages	11g
Pork chop, grilled	20g		
Small beefburger	20g		
Cheddar cheese	19g	Cottage cheese	2g
Thin-cut chips	17g	Thick-cut chips	8g
Small bar of chocolate	15g		
Minced beef	14g	Minced beef, fat poured off	6g
Edam cheese	13g		
Double cream	13g	Single cream	6g
Small bag of peanuts	12g		
Roast chicken, with skin	12g	Roast chicken, without skin	4g
Fish fingers, fried	11g	Fish fingers, grilled	6g
Halva	11g		
Small bag of crisps	11g	Fat-reduced crisps	7g
Butter or margarine	8g		
Roast potatoes	8g	Boiled or baked potatoes	0g

Cholesterol Query

Cholesterol is a soft, waxy substance that carries fat around the body and helps protect our vital organs. Despite the bad press cholesterol has received over the last few years, this is a vitally important substance in our bodies. The body makes its own supply in the bile ducts, so even if we cut out all cholesterol from our diet our body will continue to make the amount that it needs. Although high cholesterol levels have been linked to heart disease, the amount of dietary cholesterol we get from our foods has only a limited effect on our blood cholesterol levels. This means that many foods that contain cholesterol, such as eggs, offal, and shellfish, can be safely eaten. A far more important factor is the amount of saturated fat that we eat. This type of fat does raise our blood cholesterol count and the greater the level in our blood, the more at risk we become from heart disease (the biggest cause of death in the UK).

It is estimated that about two-thirds of all adults in the UK have a blood cholesterol level that is above 5.2 mmoL/L (the average target). When high cholesterol levels occur, certain oils can be useful in lowering our cholesterol score. Fish oils in the diet are important cholesterol lowerers. Vegetable oils are also useful for preventing the build-up of excess cholesterol in our arteries. Some vegetable oils, such as sunflower and olive oil, are rich in the antioxidant vitamin E, which acts as a kind of detergent on the excess cholesterol and helps to prevent it from clogging the arteries. This may be one reason why Mediterranean-style diets rich in olive oil are believed to lower the risk of heart disease. The role of vitamin E in fighting heart disease will be examined in more detail in Chapter Four.

Good vs Bad Cholesterol

Most of the cholesterol in our bloodstream is found in the form of LDLs. This stands for low-density lipoproteins. These are known as the 'bad' form of cholesterol because high levels build up in our arteries and lead to the fatty plaque deposits that are a prime cause of heart disease and strokes. By contrast, there is also a 'good' form of cholesterol called high-density lipoproteins, or HDLs. These blood fats are beneficial because they help to carry the LDL out of the arteries and prevent its long-term build up. High levels of HDL are associated with a low risk of heart disease, the number one killer of both men and women in the UK today.

Ways to Cut-back on Fat
- Switch to skimmed or semi-skimmed milk
- Use a non-stick frying pan
- Use a squirt of oil spray for frying

- Cook with vegetable stock instead of shallow frying in oil or butter
- Always trim all the visible fat from meat
- Eat more fish and poultry
- Choose lower fat cheeses, such as cottage cheese
- Use low-fat yogurt instead of evaporated milk or cream
- Steam, grill or bake whenever possible

Sugars

We are a nation of sugarholics. Confectionery sales totalling £2,332 million in 1984 were greater than the combined sum spent on bread and cereals – and the body has no need to eat any type of sugar at all! Both brown and white sugar supply only empty calories and absolutely no nourishment whatsoever. All types of sugar are also very high in calories and, after fat, are the next most powerful diet destructors. In addition to piling on the pounds, sugar has been linked to lowered immunity, diabetes and skin disorders. Too much refined sugar in our diet makes us more likely to put on weight and this in turn leads to a much greater risk of heart disease, strokes and high blood pressure. Britain's leading obesity expert, Professor John Garrow, at St Bartholomew's Hospital Medical School, London, is also convinced that it is the unusual way in which sugar is broken down by the body that is particularly significant in its link with obesity, making it more important than previously thought.

As with fat, there are many different ways to describe sugar on the labels. Some may believe that one type of sugar may be better for us than others, but the fact is that sugar, sucrose, glucose, dextrose and all the other 'oses' have no nutritional value other than feeding the body with empty worthless calories.

Sweet Nature

SUCROSE

This is the white or brown sugar used in sweets, biscuits and cakes. Sucrose comes from sugar beet and sugar cane and is itself made up of two simpler sugars called fructose and glucose.

FRUCTOSE

This is found in sugar and honey and is the sweetest tasting sugar. Fructose tastes one third sweeter than sucrose. Buying packets of refined fructose to use instead of refined sugar (sucrose) can save a third of our sugar calories as you will need to use less of it.

GLUCOSE

This is naturally found in some foods and is also known as dextrose. Glucose gives us energy but this doesn't mean that we need sweets or sports drinks with added glucose. Our energy supplies come from complex carbohydrates, or starches, which the body breaks down into simple sugars. These are then digested and absorbed as energy. As long as we get our glucose this way we do not need to eat any type of sugar at all.

LACTOSE

This is the main sugar found in milk and other dairy products and is about one third as sweet as sucrose.

MALTOSE

This sugar is manufactured from starch. As with all other sugars, the body eventually breaks it down into glucose.

Not only are sugars high in calories, but they are also low in important nutrients and do not contain any of the important ACE vitamins. In terms of our health, the most important difference between the different types of sugars are those that are locked into the structure of a food (intrinsic sugars) and those that are added (extrinsic sugars).

The intrinsic sugars can be found in the fruits and vegetables that also contain the ACE vitamins. These intrinsic sugars are not harmful to our health. Extrinsic sugars are made by processing foods to release the sugars. For example, an apple contains intrinsic sugars, but turning it into processed apple purée frees the sugars and makes them extrinsic. These 'free' sugars should be used with caution. The exception is thought to be lactose which, although it is an extrinsic sugar, is not thought to damage our health. Nutritionists talk in terms of non-milk extrinsic sugars (NME) as being the types of sugars we should especially cut down on. Remember – NME is the 'enemy' and includes all added sugars, table sugar, concentrated fruit juices and honey.

A 1993 report by the joint Department of Dental Public Health at London Hospital Medical College and University College London analysed the recommendations of 115 scientific studies on diet and health over the last 10 years. The overwhelming majority of these advised a dramatic reduction in the amount of extrinsic sugars that we eat. Intrinsic sugars in fruits were not seen to be harmful, but the amount of extrinsic sugars should only amount to less than 10 percent of our total daily calories. This figure should be even lower for those wanting to achieve successful weight-loss.

It is important to resist the advertising images that promote sugar as a health food. The sugar manufacturers Tate and Lyle and British Sugar spent around £10 million on their extensive 'hummingbird' advertising campaign. However, this blurred the important difference between extrinsic white sugar and intrinsic sugars in whole fruits. Reducing a sweet tooth is important for life-long better health. Sweets and confectionery do the body no good at all. They only contain 'empty' calories as they provide no reasonable level of basic nutrition. However, some sweets are misleadingly sold as energy-boosting snacks. True, you may feel a temporary lift in energy levels after eating a chocolate bar, but look at what really happens inside the body.

Eating a sugary snack which is 100 percent sugar means that in 10–15 minutes the blood-sugar level rises dramatically. This initial spurt of energy is quickly followed by a more lasting low. This is because insulin is secreted when blood-sugar levels are high and this stores sugar from the bloodstream into our cells. So blood-sugar levels drop and leave us feeling hungrier than before. This is not a true hunger, as we only ate the sweets initially as a quick snack, but it fools the brain into believing that the stomach is empty. Sugar not only rots the teeth but can also trigger the appetite. If you have a sweet tooth and want to eat sugar, only eat it with a meal so that the rate of absorption is slowed down. Artificial sweeteners may also stimulate the appetite by triggering the release of gastric juices in the stomach in the anticipation of a raised blood-glucose level. Hunger pangs may then follow as the sweeteners fail to provide any of the expected calories. For this reason it is also best only to eat chemical sweeteners at meal times.

Better still, follow these points to reduce sugar cravings:

- Gradually cut down the amount of sugar you use in drinks and sprinkle on cereals until you stop altogether
- Always keep a supply of fruit nearby to snack on
- Seedless white grapes are the sweetest fruits and will satisfy the worst sugar cravings
- A daily supplement of the mineral dolomite may help reduce sugar cravings
- Buy reduced or no-sugar versions of foods and drinks
- Sweet brown rice (from health-food shops) is naturally rich in intrinsic sugars and makes a great rice pudding.
- Dried fruits are high in calories because they contain concentrated fruit sugars, but a handful of raisins is better for you than a sugary snack
- Carrots are also rich in natural sugars, so keep carrot sticks in the fridge for when you feel like snacking
- When cooking, cut the amount of sugar in a recipe by at least half. You will never need as much as recipes quote
- Never, ever give sugary foods or drinks to babies
- Beware of ingredients ending in 'ose' such as sucrose, dextrose etc. and of any syrups such as corn syrup.

Although the amount of packet sugar we buy has almost halved in the last decade, we are still eating *more* of the white stuff. This is due to the switch from home baking to convenience foods and confectionery. Most of the sugars we now eat come from processed foods and drinks, such as sweetened fruit juices and cans of fizzy drinks. When buying foods that contain sugars, always check the labels first. Ingredients must be listed in order, with the greatest first. But by dividing sugar into many different types, such as dextrose, maltose and glucose, manufacturers can make sure it will appear lower down the list. When these different types are added together, you may find that sugar is actually the main ingredient. Foods described as having 'no added sugar' or 'unsweetened' are not necessarily low in sugar. They could be foods that are naturally high in sugar or may be sweetened with concentrated fruit juices (extrinsic sugars). Food labels are often a complicated maze of weasel-words and misinformation. Check out the labels in your shopping trolley and see how many actually contain sugar as the main ingredient.

Teaspoons of Sugar

Aim for less than six teaspoons of NME sugars a day.
(Remember the body does not actually need any at all.)
(1 level teaspoon = 5g sugar, 1 sugar lump = 2.5g)

Food	Quantity	Teaspoons
Mars bar	regular size (65g)	8.5
Coca Cola	1 can (330ml)	7.0
Danish pastry	1 (110g)	6.5
Lucozade	small bottle (250ml)	4.5
Sugar Puffs	1 bowl (40g)	4.0
Unsweetened orange juice	1 carton (200ml)	3.5
Baked beans	small tin (205g)	2.5
Tinned spaghetti	small tin (215g)	2.0

Artificial Sweeteners

As adding refined sugar to foods is to be avoided, are artificial sweeteners the solution to the problem? No. It is far better to retrain your taste buds to accept fewer sweet foods than to become dependent on a packet of chemicals.

Britons spend around £50 million a year on artificial sweeteners, so sugar substitutes are clearly a big business. Although they provide all the sweetness of sugar with none of the calories, there is a sour note about their safety. While most scientific studies have passed artificial sweeteners for safety, many critics believe that there is still a cause for concern. For example, some studies show that saccharin may increase the risk of cancer and cyclamates have been banned from most European countries. In America, foods containing saccharin even carry a printed warning that it may be 'hazardous to your health'. The use of artificial sweeteners in processed foods has been growing at an alarming rate in recent years. Four out of five children have saccharin at least once a week, usually in the form of soft drinks and squashes. The UK allows manufacturers to add artificial sweeteners to foods and drinks together with refined sugar. This means that you or your child could be eating large amounts of these chemicals even if there is no 'diet' label on the product.

So what really goes into these handy-sized boxes of small white pills? Artificial sweeteners are essentially a cocktail of chemicals. The formula on a typical well-known brand reads like the contents of a chemistry set: sodium bicarbonate, trisodium citrate, saccharin, sodium carbonate, glycine and monosodium glutamate. No wonder they don't label the ingredients on the packet – it isn't big enough!

Most artificial sweeteners are known in the food industry as *intense sweeteners*. This group contains the chemicals aspartame, acesulfame-K, cyclamates, thaumatin and saccharin. All of these are classified as food additives. The food industry may also use another group called *bulk sweeteners*, which include sorbitol, mannitol, lacitol, xylitol and isomalt. These are actually 'sweet' alcohols or polyols and naturally occur in fruit. These bulk sweeteners are also commercially produced by combining sugars such as glucose and lactose with hydrogen to harden them (in a similar way to hydrogenated fats). Their only real advantage over ordinary sugar is that they will not contribute to tooth decay, although they do contain just as many calories. I'm afraid there is no alternative but to wean yourself off sugar and its substitutes as much as possible. You don't have to cut all sugar out of your life overnight, but start reducing the amount you eat now – grain by grain, if necessary.

Full of Fibre

You can see from the ACE Plan Pyramid on page 17 that eating plenty of carbohydrates is the basis for your new weight-loss regime. Carbohydrates are good guys because the body stores any extra carbohydrate we eat in the form of glycogen. The body cannot make much glycogen from fatty foods. This means that the body resists making extra fat from carbohydrates until its glycogen stores are replenished.

● *It is very hard for the body to turn carbohydrates into fat.*

Regular exercise means that an extra helping of pasta is unlikely to end up as fat layers on our hips and thighs. When our carbohydrate consumption drops, so do our glycogen stores. Several pounds of water are stored along with the glycogen and these are the pounds that are lost when we stop eating carbohydrates. This small amount of weight-loss looks great on the scales, but it does not mean much in the long term. Unfortunately, the loss of a few pounds of water does not represent any real loss of excess body fat.

All nutritionists agree that one of the most important rules of any weight-loss or healthy eating plan is to eat *much* more in the way of carbohydrates because they are packed with fibre. One of the many reasons why the *Weight-Loss for Life* menus work is because they focus on high-fibre carbohydrates that enable us to feel full on fewer calories. High-fibre foods also tend to be low in fat and sugar – another good reason why they are the perfect partner for successful slimming. The bottom line is that we all need fibre. Too little fibre in our daily diet results in the bowels becoming sluggish and constipated. This then leads to further problems such as varicose veins, gallstones and piles. In the longer term, a low-fibre diet increases the risk of colon cancer as the body is unable to eliminate toxins effectively and speedily.

Unfortunately, the average diet has dramatically changed during the last decade. We are eating far more processed foods such as white bread, refined fats and sugars than ever before. We have given up our previous dietary staples, including oats, barley and lentils in favour of low-fibre, convenience foods. By contrast, those living in Mediterranean countries such as Spain and Italy have continued to eat the same foods for thousands of years. The Southern Europeans eat many more fresh fruits, vegetables and whole grains in the form of breads and pasta. This has resulted in a much lower incidence of chronic disease, such as heart disease and cancer. Fibre provides the broom to give our insides a thorough sweep and cleans out the colon where some of the most dangerous diseases breed. Eating more fibre is important, not only for long-term weight-loss but also for better health, increased vitality and energy levels.

Adding fibre-rich foods to our everyday meals is simple, inexpensive and very easy. Whole-grain cereals provide about ten times as much fibre as ordinary cornflakes, so a simple switch in your breakfast bowl can dramatically boost your fibre intake. Adding a spoonful of pot barley to soups or eating potatoes with their (scrubbed) skins also makes the most of the natural fibre in cheap, plentiful foods. Eating refined grains such as white flour, however, does not work so well. This is because these have had the outer husk stripped away during food processing. Not only does this remove our fibre, it also leaches away the valuable vitamin E found in the fibrous husk or 'germ' of wheat. Refined white flour contains less than a quarter of the vitamin E found in wholemeal flour and has about a fifth of its magnesium and zinc content. Refined flour is not only a poor source of one of the essential ACE vitamins, it is also remarkably low in fibre.

Fibre Facts

Wholemeal bread and whole grains are probably the first thing we think of as being high in fibre. But the ACE vitamin-rich fruits and vegetables are also some of our very best sources. Fibre is basically a carbohydrate that is broken down in the intestine and it comes in several different guises. It consists of the cellulose fibres that form the structure of green, leafy vegetables and the outer skins of sweetcorn and beans. There are two types of fibre: soluble fibre, which is soft and spongy and insoluble fibre, which is coarse and hard. Soluble fibre is essential for successful weight-loss as it dissolves in the liquids in the stomach and helps to fill us up and prevent hunger pangs. Soluble fibre is also important in the upper portion of the gut where it slows down the absorption of nutrients from food. This is no bad thing, as it allows time for the vital ACE vitamins to work their way into the bloodstream before the food passes into the colon. Soluble fibre is also vital for regulating the release of glucose into the bloodstream. This means we avoid hunger pangs and sudden sugar cravings as our blood sugars are stabilized. The best way to avoid an attack of the 'munchies' is to make sure we eat plenty of soluble fibre from fruits, vegetables, oats and oatmeal.

By contrast, insoluble fibre has only one main function: to expel waste matter from the body. Insoluble fibre is found in the husks of whole grains, such as brown rice and wholewheat foods. Unlike soluble fibre, this does not dissolve inside the stomach, but passes through the digestive system more or less intact. The job of insoluble fibre is to bind with toxins and waste matter in the system and expel them in faeces. Too little insoluble fibre in our daily diet not only causes constipation, but also means that the poisons the body needs to get rid of daily lurk in our insides for longer. We need to make sure that we eat large amounts of both soluble and insoluble fibre every day of our lives. This will speed weight-loss by reducing our appetite. It will also boost our energy levels by speeding the removal of toxins from the system that conspire to make us feel tired and lethargic.

Fibre Providers

Raw bran is not very tasty to eat. The other problems with unprocessed bran is that it contains substances called phytates which bind with iron, zinc and calcium. Phytates prevent these important minerals from being absorbed and used by the body. ACE vitamin-rich foods are a much better option. One tablespoon of raw bran gives you 2.5g of fibre – yuk! But the following provide the same amount, plus some of the ACE vitamins and are a much more appetising option:

- 25 raspberries
- 20 strawberries
- 15 blackberries
- 8 sprouts
- 6 dates
- 5 dried apricots
- 4 tablespoons of cooked lentils
- 3 dried figs
- 2 bananas
- 2 slices of brown bread
- 2 kiwi fruit
- 1 slice of wholemeal bread
- 1 wholemeal scone or muffin
- 1 orange, large apple or nectarine
- 1 small bag of nuts and raisins
- half a jacket potato
- half a pear
- half a bowl of muesli
- quarter of a mango

Labelling Lore

Although much of our food labelling system has yet to be perfected, the labels printed on the sides of cartons, bottles, packets, cans and jars reveal a good deal about their contents. Here's what to look out for when you want the healthiest options for you and your family.

100g gives you:		
Energy	1400 kJ/	Kilojoules are an alternative measure of energy
	340 kcal	Kcals indicates how many calories (a measure of energy) are in each 100 g (4 oz) serving
Protein	13.8 g	
Carbohydrates	68.8 g	Carbohydrates include sugars.
of which sugars	7.2 g	We should cut down on sugars and eat more *starch*. In this case, most of the carbohydrates are starch, which is a good sign.
Fat	5.2 g	The fat content is divided into saturated and non-saturated fats. Saturated fats should be avoided. Here, the fat content is mostly unsaturated, so it is a healthier option. However, the fat content of all foods should be limited.
of which saturates	0.8 g	
Sodium	0.6 g	Sodium means salt. Choose low sodium foods.
Fibre	14.6 g	This food gives you nearly half the daily target of 30 gms

3
FITNESS VERSUS FATNESS

It's not the years in your life – but the life in
your years that counts

Regular exercise is the key to renewed energy and vitality. It also gives the body the key to unlock the fat stored in our fat cells. For this to happen, we need to supply the body with oxygen in the form of aerobic exercise. The term aerobic means 'with oxygen' and covers any form of sustained exercise that makes us breathe harder, so we take in deep gulps of oxygen. Aerobic exercise is very easy and does not require any special equipment, expensive gym membership or facilities. Brisk walking is an excellent form of aerobic exercise – provided that it is fast enough to leave you puffing. Running up the stairs is also a good at-home version of the more expensive 'stepper'machines that the good gyms are now equipped with. However, all aerobic exercise must be maintained for a minimum of *twenty minutes* for the body to benefit. This means that stop/start activities such as golf, cricket and gymnastics do not strictly qualify as 'aerobic' because they do not produce a steady increase in the heart rate needed over a twenty-minute period to release fat from cells.

How active are you?

Discover your daily activity fitness score with this simple quiz. Keep track of your progress by repeating the quiz each month and comparing the score. See how fast your level increases!

Weekday Walking
(e.g. to and from work, school or shopping) Score
None	0
15-20 minutes a day	1
20-40 minutes a day	2
40-60 minutes a day	3
More than 60 minutes a day	4

Active Chores
(e.g. gardening, housework, washing the car etc.) Score
None	0
Fairly inactive	1
Up to 4 hours a week	2
4-8 hours a week	3
More than 8 hours a week	4

Vigorous Exercise
(e.g. sports, jogging, up-hill cycling, swimming, heavy manual work, gym sessions) Score
None	0
Less than once a week	1
Once or twice a week	2
Two or three times a week	3
More than three times a week	4

Score 0-2
You are a real couch-potato and extremely inactive. Get up and do something with your body before it seizes up altogether!

Score 3-4
You are fairly active but need to take more planned exercise to raise your metabolism and burn fat faster

Score 5-6
You are an active person with a good level of physical activity. Make sure you take some form of planned exercise every other day to keep your activity routine constant.

Score 7-12
You are extremely active and physically fit. Make sure you vary your activities so that each of your different muscle groups benefits. You would do well to take a vitamin E supplement to reduce muscle fatigue and protect cells from the increased free radical activity caused by vigorous exercise.

The human body was designed for regular exercise and gentle exertion over long periods of time. It is only in today's sedentary age of the car, computer and washing machine that we are under-utilizing our own physical capabilities. Exercise is well worth the effort as it actually increases our energy levels – it won't wear you out, it will make you *more* energetic! Regular exercise increases the enzymes that help the body burn up the fats and sugars in our food. In many cases, the problem of being overweight has less to do with too much fat and more to do with too little active muscle. Improving our muscle-tone means we also improve our ability to burn up calories as the mechanics of the body become more efficient.

Developing muscle tissue doesn't make us bigger though. Muscle-toning through exercise means your zips will zip up and your buttons fasten without bulging. This is far more important than the reading on your scales. The figures on the scales can be very misleading. For example, a lean athlete may actually weigh more than a chubby couch-potato. We need to increase muscle weight, not decrease it.

Calorie Counter	
Exercise	Approx. Kcals per hour
Step aerobics	600
Jumping rope	600
Aerobics	550
Swimming	500
Tennis	450
Cycling	400
Badminton	350
Fast walking	300

Stamina Sessions

The benefit of regular exercising is that it increases stamina. This means that you are able to perform physical tasks for longer without feeling the strain. In addition to strength and suppleness, stamina is a useful measurement of our overall fitness and helps determine how quickly we burn up our calories in the form of fuel. Try this simple stamina test each month to monitor your fitness progress. If you are exercising for at least twenty minutes, three times a week, you will find that your stamina levels quickly increase. Keep a record in your diary – and watch your personal fitness levels soar!

Step 1: Choose a safe, flat route about a mile long (check the distance on a map or with a car milometer).

Step 2: Put on a pair of comfortable walking shoes or trainers.

Step 3: Walking, running (or a combination of the two) see how long it takes you to complete the distance of one mile.

Step 4: Compare your time with the chart opposite. Keep a note of your time and see how much it improves over the months to come.

Minutes per mile	Stamina fitness
20 or more	very unfit
15 – 20	unfit
12 – 15	fair
10 – 12	fit
10 or under	very fit

Finding the Time to Exercise

- The main hurdle to overcome is to START EXERCIS-ING. The only way you will find out how good it feels is to make a start.
- Take one day at a time. Every day try a little more activity. Get off the bus one stop earlier, walk to the newsagents, take the dog for a run instead of a walk, take the stairs and not the lift. Each one of these simple steps increases your energy capacity and helps burn off excess fat.
- Don't try and do too much in life. If you are too busy to exercise, you are just TOO BUSY!
- Keep a record of your exercising. Make a wall chart in the kitchen or office and fill in the days you exercise, or keep a note in your diary. Try and take some form of vigorous exercise *at least* three times each week.
- Be persistent with your body – don't ever give up. If you feel too tired to work out one day, set aside time in the evening to go through some simple stretches in-stead. Make up for any lost exercising by doing a little more the following day.
- Be realistic with your exercise goals. Failure is no fun, so be kind to yourself by setting achievable targets.
- Use your time effectively. Look at ways to save time during the day that could be better spent taking some form of exercise.
- Regular exercise is a great de-stresser as it loosens physical tension in the body and clears the mind. Vigorous exercise also produces brain chemicals that

48

encourage feelings of well-being. Get yourself hooked on that natural high!

- Remember in the final analysis, nothing has a higher priority in life than your personal health and well-being. You can only achieve this by regular, vigorous exercise.

ACE Exercise

Children

It is important to introduce children to the idea of taking some form of regular exercise while still young. This will help them to maintain a lithe, lean figure as they grow up and prevent them from developing into lazy, fat adults. Lifestyle routines established now will become the habits of a lifetime. However, it is important not to emphasize the weight-loss advantages to young children. You can score an own-goal by making youngsters unhealthily paranoid about their appearance. Instead of stressing weight-loss, highlight the benefits of health and fitness gain. Children will also benefit from improved hand to eye co-ordination and the philosophies of teamwork, co-operation, self-improvement and self-esteem.

Exercise during childhood is doubly important as it stimulates healthy bone development. Fun activities such as obstacle courses, kite-flying and games of tag are good for encouraging movement in toddlers and younger children. Older children can be introduced to team-games and sports. Teenagers and young children should not do too much weight-training to develop their muscles as this can stunt bone growth. Excessive weight-training and resistance exercises should be avoided before eighteen to twenty years of age. This is the age when the epiphyseal plates seal the tops of our bones with a lattice-work layer to prevent any further growth. Load-bearing exercises can damage the formation of these structures and lead to bone and joint problems in later life. Excessive exercise during puberty can also play havoc with the female menstrual cycle and delay the onset of, or disrupt, periods. It may

49

even stop them altogether (a disorder known as amenor-rhoea).

Adults
All adults need regular exercise. This is not only important for successful weight-loss, but also for better health, stamina and mobility. The best form of exercise is one which leaves you feeling breathless, but that you can sustain for twenty minutes or more. The following are all good forms of aerobic exercise.
- jogging
- brisk walking
- swimming
- aerobic classes
- rebounding on a mini-trampoline
- step exercises in a class or with a video
- roller skating
- team games such as hockey, netball, football etc.

In order for aerobic exercise to release fat from our cells it needs to be sustained for at least 20 minutes, for a minimum of three times each week. During these periods of aerobic exercise, we need to raise our pulse to within the fat releasing Target Heart Rate. Each one of us has a slightly different Target Heart Rate and you can find your personal fat releasing THR by following this simple formula:

220 minus your age $\times$ 60% = low Target Heart Rate
220 minus your age $\times$ 75% = high Target Heart Rate

Target Heart Rates decrease with age and are lowered by one beat per minute every year. The average fat releasing target band is between 110 and 140 beats per minute. In order for an exercise routine to reduce fat, you will need to raise your pulse to a level between the upper and lower target rate. Remember, if you get bored with exercising, change it! Join a keep-fit group, take up a sport, go jogging with the children, buy a dog! However, do be aware that increasing the amount of oxygen we breathe in also increases the levels of potentially damaging free radicals. The answer is to eat more of the antioxidant ACE vitamins to protect our cells. This is especially important if you exercise outside where you may be breathing in high levels of toxic pollutants, such as car exhaust fumes. If you have any medical condition or are taking any medication you should obtain your GP's approval before commencing any intensive exercise routine.

This chart gives you an at-a-glance guide to your Target Heart Range (THR)

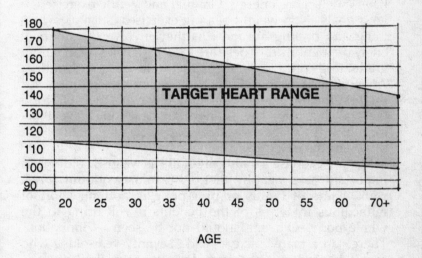

AGE

As you begin exercising, aim for the low range of your Target Heart Rate. When you become physically fitter, increase the range to the upper end of the scale. The fitter you are, the higher your THR.

The Elderly
Old age is no obstacle to exercise and there is no reason why we should not continue to be active as we grow older. Many of our bodily functions go into decline over the age

of 60, so we have all the more reason to keep ourselves fit and active. Once we are past the age of 60 our metabolic rate drops so we burn calories less efficiently. Our maximal (greatest possible) heart rate reduces as our heart ages, our muscle strength reduces and our bone mineral mass also declines. For these reasons it is important to take it slow and steady when starting any exercise regime.

If it is many years since you took any regular, planned form of exercise, or if you have gained a great deal of weight in recent years, it is going to take a little time before you notice the benefits of exercise. However, with time and perseverance you will feel fitter, more mobile and have much more energy. Gradual and gentle exercise are your goals. Non-weight bearing exercises, such as swimming and cycling are ideal as they involve the minimal energy expenditure. These are a good starting point before graduating onto a more structured exercise routine. Anyone considering starting an exercise programme for the first time in a few years should consult their GP for a medical check-up. This is important as it could reveal factors such as diabetes and osteoporosis which may not otherwise be detected.

Making exercise a daily part of life as we grow older is as important as a healthy diet. A regular work-out, brisk walk, game of tennis or ping-pong is nothing short of miraculous in terms of the benefits it will bring to the whole body. Old age should not be seen as limitation. There are many sixty- and seventy-year-olds who regularly work out at a gym. Even those in their nineties can make significant improvements in their muscle strength. At the Human Nutrition Research Center in Boston, USA, men and women in their eighties and nineties are frequently put through strenuous exercise programmes and weight-lifting circuits to improve their overall health and wellbeing. Age is more a state of mind and body than a chronological fact of life. An active seventy-year-old can be fitter and have more stamina than a sedentary thirty-year-old. The best advice to anyone in their later years is to stay active. Those who have let their activity level slip should start a slow, progressive exercise programme based on low-impact activities such as walking, exercising machines in a gym, yoga and keep-fit classes.

Although walking is a weight-bearing activity it is also a good form of exercise. You should always increase your duration of walking before increasing the intensity or pace. Before taking any form of exercise it is well worth completing a gentle warm-up routine. This should include stretches to mobilize the joints and muscles and will improve mobility and flexibility. Stretching before taking exercise also reduces the risk of injury as it prepares the body for activity by boosting the blood circulation and raising the heart rate for aerobic benefits. For a stretch to be really effective, hold it still for ten to fifteen seconds (without bouncing) before releasing. Always hold onto the back of a stable chair or table to avoid overbalancing. A few simple stretches after completing any form of exercise also reduces the risk of stiff muscles and future injury.

Fluid Replacement

No matter what our age, we all need to drink plenty of water while we exercise. Drinking water to rehydrate the system allows the body to function effectively and enables us to work out harder. Even a couch-potato needs to drink around two litres of water a day. This level increases dramatically during hot weather and during exercise. In the hot, humid summer months the body may need as much as ten litres a day to maintain the status quo. During periods of intense exercise we sweat up to two litres of water per hour and this fluid needs to be replaced. Drink small amounts of water during exercise and drink it frequently. Avoid drinking caffeine drinks (coffee, tea and cola drinks) shortly before, during, or one hour after exercise as caffeine is a diuretic and encourages water loss. If you feel thirsty your body probably dehydrated twenty minutes ago. This is especially important for pregnant women and the elderly.

TWELVE GOOD REASONS WHY YOU SHOULD EXERCISE:

- Exercise burns off the calories you would otherwise store as fat

- Exercise strengthens and slims the body

- Exercise increases bone density, flexibility and improves posture

- Exercise reduces the risk of heart disease, cancer and back pain

- Exercise helps you to relax and unwind, and reduces tension

- Exercise increases everyday energy levels

- Exercise helps to reduce your appetite temporarily

- Exercise boosts your metabolic rate – even when resting

- Exercise improves the appearance of cellulite

- Exercise stimulates the lymphatic system, keeps the skin clear and the immune system strong

- Exercise improves your sex life!

- Exercise slows down the ageing process and keeps you young

4

THE ROLE OF ACE VITAMINS

'We are opening up a whole new frontier for vitamins'

Professor Jialal, University of Texas

A few years ago the word 'antioxidant' and 'free radical' were not in your vocabulary unless you happened to be a biochemist. Outside the rarefied world of research chemistry it is only recently that the scientific connections have been made to link the three vitamins A, C and E together as a group of unique nutrients. Collectively they are known as antioxidant nutrients and they have the power to prevent chronic diseases.

Each of the ACE vitamins has a unique role to play in health, well-being and life-long weight-loss. The ACE super-slim foods are the fruits, vegetables and whole grains that contain high levels of the special antioxidant nutrients, vitamin A (in the form of beta-carotene), vitamin C and vitamin E.

Vitamins are essential substances that act in various important ways to keep us fit and healthy. We cannot do without vitamins and if we don't get enough we can become ill and even die of a vitamin deficiency. The most important antioxidant nutrients in everyday foods are beta-carotene, vitamin C and vitamin E. Other useful nutrients with antioxidant properties are the minerals selenium, copper, manganese and zinc. In addition, there are a newly recognized group of trace nutrients present in fruits and vegetables called flavonoids. We will take a closer look at these a little later in this chapter.

Why are the ACE vitamins so important?

Beta-carotene, vitamin C and vitamin E are known in nutritional jargon as antioxidants. This means that they fight against the process of oxidation that occurs inside the body. Scientists are now recognizing the importance of this when it comes to growing old and developing serious diseases. On a day-to-day level these vitamins are essential for keeping the body fit, healthy and energetic. We can see the results of oxidation all around us in everyday life. For example, if you slice up an apple and leave it for half an hour the inside quickly turns brown, because the apple is reacting with oxygen in the air. Similarly, a car chassis will rust when left outside for long periods of time because it is exposed to oxygen in the atmosphere. An identical process is taking place within our bodies every second of our lives. Although we can't see what's going on, our body is literally 'rusting' from within, due to this continual process of oxidation and the action of damaging free radicals.

The ACE vitamins and minerals that help to keep us youthful, fit and healthy are nature's answer to the damage caused by oxidation. Each of these nutrients acts in a slightly different way, but their overall effect is to mop up the free radicals as they form and prevent them from going on to do serious damage within the body. As free radicals are continually being created, it is well worth maintaining high levels of each of these vital vitamins. In addition, many nutrients are involved with the important process of energy creation within the body. This is a vital element of maintaining a healthy metabolism and burning calories, leading to long-term permanent weight-loss.

The Free Radical Factor

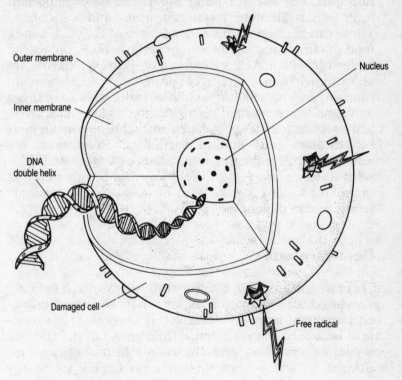

Outer membrane

Inner membrane

DNA double helix

Nucleus

Damaged cell

Free radical

ACE Weight-loss

The principles of *Weight-Loss for Life* focus on eating ACE-vitamin enriched foods to boost the metabolism, provide the body with the best sources of energy and concentrate on vital low-fat and healthful foods. ACE eating for weight-loss is based on eating plenty of complex carbo-hydrates daily. As we have seen from the ACE eating pyramid on page 17, this means between five and nine portions *every day* of a carbohydrate food, such as wholemeal bread, brown rice, wheat germ, pasta, pulses, beans and lentils. Many of these ACE super-slimming foods contain valuable vitamin E and all are high in fibre and other nutrients, but low in fat and sugar. The other important ACE super-slimming foods are fruits and vegetables. These can be seen on the second layer of the ACE eating food pyramid, and are important because they contain the highest levels of ACE vitamins. For example, carrots are an extremely rich source of beta-carotene (which the body can convert into vitamin A), citrus fruits such as oranges and lemons are bursting with vitamin C, while dark green leafy vegetables such as spinach and cabbage contain both beta-carotene and vitamin C, with small amounts of vitamin E. To realize the huge significance of these ACE vitamins in terms of overall weight-loss and health gain it is important to look at how each of these special nutrients works inside the body.

Beta-carotene

This nutrient works in two very different ways. It is firstly converted into vitamin A by the body and the left-over part functions as an antioxidant. It is important not to confuse beta-carotene with actual vitamin A, as the two are separate substances; vitamin A is not technically an antioxidant. It was one of the earliest vitamins to be discovered. A lack of vitamin A is still the number one cause of blindness in underdeveloped countries today. It was officially identified in 1913 by American researchers and there are two main types. One is found in foods but comes from animal sources, such as meat and milk, and this form is called retinol. The other versions of vitamin A are the carotenoids that are found in fruit and vegetables. There are around 600 of these, but the most important one for us is beta-carotene. The body is able to convert beta-carotene into vitamin A as it needs it, which explains why vegetarians manage to get all the vitamin A they need without eating any animal produce.

Vitamin A is a fat-soluble nutrient and so is only found in fatty parts of food. It is present in meat (especially liver, where the animal stores its supplies of vitamin A) and in dairy products such as milk, butter and cheese. Fish liver oils are one of the richest natural sources of vitamin A, which is one reason why a daily spoonful of cod liver oil does the body so much good. But as with other fat-soluble nutrients, if we eat too much vitamin A, it ends up being stored in our own liver, which is why eating large quantities of this vitamin can cause liver damage and is toxic. Although large quantities of vitamin A are not advised and may be dangerous, the equivalent amount of beta-carotene is totally safe. It is almost impossible to take too much beta-carotene as the body only converts it into the amount of vitamin A that it actually needs. Not only is beta-carotene non-toxic, it is also a powerful antioxidant that combats a particularly potent oxygen radical called singlet oxygen. This makes it a preferable and altogether more exciting nutrient, for the reasons we shall now discover.

What is Beta-carotene?
Beta-carotene is a natural plant pigment and was first discovered in carrots, hence its name. Scientists first became interested in beta-carotene over 150 years ago. However it is only relatively recently that the full exciting potential of beta-carotene has been explored.

Pure beta-carotene is a deep shade of reddish orange and is one of the main pigments in yellow- and orange-coloured fruits and vegetables. Foods rich in beta-carotene are easy to find as they stand out on the supermarket shelves in bright colours, for example carrots and mangoes. In general, the riper the produce, the more beta-carotene it contains. Green leafy vegetables are also rich in beta-carotene although they are a different colour because the dark green chlorophyll pigment is more dominant. The darker and more vivid the colour of the fruit or vegetable the more beta-carotene it contains. This is why dark lettuce leaves contain more beta-carotene than the pale iceberg variety.

In addition to the benefits of beta-carotene being converted into vitamin A, the nutrient is now being studied for its other exciting property, namely as one of our most powerful antioxidants. The role of beta-carotene in plants is to help prevent fruits and vegetables from frazzling in the sun. This is an antioxidant action as it protects the plants from the free radicals generated by sunlight. Beta-carotene has a similar effect in humans and even helps prevent sun-induced skin cancers. Not only does it protect us from the free radicals generated by sunlight, but it is also one of our most effective weapons against general free radical cell damage.

Some of the most exciting research in recent years has concerned beta-carotene and its function as an anti-cancer nutrient. Cancer is still one of our major killers. This disease kills more than 160,000 Britons every year and affects every family in the land at some point in our lives. While the medical world continues its search for cures for many different types of cancer, nutritionists believe that a far easier option is preventing the disease from happening in the first place. Although we don't know exactly how or why cancer strikes, it has been shown that populations who eat the most beta-carotene in the form of fresh fruit and vegetables (for example many of the Mediterranean countries) have a greatly reduced risk of many different types of cancer.

Scientists worldwide now believe that eating a large quantity of fruits and vegetables on a daily basis will provide sufficient beta-carotene to give us significant protection against developing cancer in the future. Although the evidence is still mounting, it has sparked major trials involving beta-carotene around the world. One such study involves 23,000 physicians in America who are taking antioxidant supplements on a daily basis to see if the rate of cancer and heart disease can be lowered. Of course, fruits and vegetables are also every dieter's best friend and continue to be a vitally important part of every weight-loss regime.

Cancer Studies

As far back as 1981, the eminent professors Sir Richard Doll and Richard Peto were attributing 35 percent of all cancer to dietary factors. These include fat intake, nitrite levels in smoked meats and low levels of the antioxidant ACE nutrients. Since then, beta-carotene (together with vitamin C and vitamin E) has emerged as one of the most exciting potential cancer preventors. The reason behind beta-carotene's success at preventing cancer seems to be that it is especially good at blocking the harmful cell damage caused by unstable particles of singlet oxygen. When these damage cells within the body, cancer is more likely to occur. Beta-carotene is able to mop up the energy of up to 1,000 molecules of highly reactive singlet oxygen with one single molecule of beta-carotene.

There have been more than fifty studies of the beneficial effects of beta-carotene on cancer, involving tens of thousands of people worldwide. Since the publication of *Liz Earle's ACE Plan*, which examines the evidence for the exciting health benefits of the ACE vitamins in greater detail, many more cancer studies involving beta-carotene have been completed.

One such study by researchers in New Jersey, USA was published in *Cancer Causes and Control* in 1993. This confirmed that beta-carotene is useful in reducing cases of lung cancer. This study looked not only at the role of beta-carotene, but also the other carotenoids which are from the same chemical family. The researchers found that the carotenoids present in colourful fruits and vegetables are potent antioxidants and may react with a carcinogen in cigarette smoke to protect us against cancers in smokers. The study revealed that both men and women benefit equally and the best vegetables are yellow and green in colour (notably pumpkin and sweet potato) while the most protective fruits are coloured yellow or orange (such as apricots and mangos).

Beta-carotene Counter

Beta-carotene is measured in micrograms (mcg) and milligrams (mg). There are 1,000mcg to 1mg. Unlike vitamin A, there is no known toxicity from taking too much beta-carotene (although an excessive amount of this natural pigment can temporarily turn the skin orange!). Some of the most important medical studies from different parts of the world are now suggesting that we need to aim for a minimum of 15,000mcgs (15mg) a day. This level can only be achieved in our diet by eating *at least* five generous portions of fruit and vegetables every day. Not only will this be good for our health and well-being, this is also an important element in our work towards total weight-loss. Not only do fruit and vegetables fill us up with relatively few calories, few grams of fat and no extrinsic sugars, but they are also bursting with ACE nutrients. This is especially important in maintaining energy levels and boosting the metabolism. If you are unable to achieve a regular daily intake of 15mg of beta-carotene from a large quantity of fruits and vegetables then an additional beta-carotene supplement is worth considering. This could be especially important for children, adolescents and the elderly, all of whom tend to eat fewer fruits and vegetables.

Ten top sources of beta-carotene		
Food	mg of beta-carotene per 100g	Kcals per 100g
Carrots	4,425	35
Sweet potatoes	4,040	87
Spinach	3,840	25
Watercress/spring greens	2,270	22
Cantaloupe melon	1,000	19
Tomatoes	640	17
Asparagus	530	25
Broccoli	475	33
Apricots	405	31
Peaches	58	33

Beta-carotene is a plant pigment, so the darker and more colourful the fruits and vegetables, the more beta-carotene they contain.

Quantities of fruit and vegetables needed to provide 15mg of Beta-Carotene

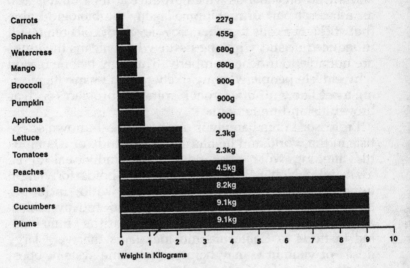

	Weight
Carrots	227g
Spinach	455g
Watercress	680g
Mango	680g
Broccoli	900g
Pumpkin	900g
Apricots	900g
Lettuce	2.3kg
Tomatoes	2.3kg
Peaches	4.5kg
Bananas	8.2kg
Cucumbers	9.1kg
Plums	9.1kg

Weight in Kilograms

Source: Boots Micronutrients Information Service

Vitamin C

This is probably the best known of all vitamins and it is the one many of us turn to when attempting to ward off the common cold. Vitamin C has been shown to have many extraordinary properties, but the bottom line is that it is absolutely essential for keeping us alive. Without enough vitamin C in our diet we are at risk from infections and may even die from scurvy.

Chemically speaking, vitamin C is one of the simplest vitamins, which is why it was among the first to be studied. Yet although it was officially identified over seventy years ago, scientists are still unravelling the mysteries of this extraordinary nutrient. Its basic function is to help with the growth and repair of body tissues and to maintain healthy gums, blood vessels, bones and teeth. It is also involved with the immune system and may be able to fight off bacteria and viral infections.

Vitamin C is mainly stored within the brain, the lungs and the adrenal glands which produce adrenalin. It is also an essential part of making collagen, the biological glue that sticks our cells together. Low levels of collagen result in reduced elasticity in lung tissue which means the lungs are not able to function properly. This may be one reason why elderly people who are likely to be low in vitamin C are more likely to suffer from respiratory problems such as bronchitis and pneumonia.

Professor Linus Pauling is one of the best-known scientists in the world and he has made the study of vitamin C his life-long work. The only single individual to be awarded a Nobel Prize twice, he also holds forty-eight honorary doctorates from around the world, including those from Oxford, Cambridge and London Universities. At ninety-three years of age, he still heads the Linus Pauling Institute in California and maintains that very large doses of vitamin C may help our immune system, boost our resistance to viruses and play a part in preventing heart disease. Although Linus Pauling's controversial theories of taking mega-doses of vitamin C to combat disease have not yet been accepted by the medical and scientific community at large, there is no doubt that vitamin C does play an important part in protecting our health.

Vitamin C has most recently hit the headlines as one of our most powerful antioxidant nutrients. As with beta-carotene, it controls and neutralizes damaging free radicals. However, unlike beta-carotene, vitamin C is water-soluble and is therefore found in the fluids that flow in between our cells. In effect, vitamin C acts as a roaming foot soldier, fighting the free radicals that cross its path as it travels throughout the body. As it is not stored within the body we need to eat foods that are rich in vitamin C as any excess simply passes through the body and is excreted in urine. The only side effect of large quantities of vitamin C (upwards of 3,000mg or 3g daily) might be mild diarrhoea. The vitamin C researchers call this 'bowel intolerance' and it varies from person to person. Interestingly, when we are fit and healthy we may only need a few grams of vitamin C before experiencing 'bowel intolerance' whereas when we are suffering from a cold or more serious disease we are able to tolerate many grams of vitamin C before rushing to the loo. Tests shows that the 'bowel intolerance' of cancer and AIDS patients may be as high as 20–30g of vitamin C a day. This indicates that the body may use extra vitamin C in some unknown way when we are unwell.

Because it is an antioxidant and water-soluble, vitamin C acts as a natural food preservative by preventing the rancidity caused by free radicals. Also known as ascorbic acid, vitamin C is often used by the food industry as an additive to foods such as cakes and biscuits. However these are not foods that feature heavily in this book! Fruits and vegetables are a far better natural source of vitamin C. Potatoes eaten with their skins are a good source of vitamin C and being carbohydrates, are also useful for a weight-loss regime. The best way to cook potatoes to maximize their vitamin content and minimize their fat level is to boil them in their skins or to bake them in their jackets. Other easily obtainable sources of vitamin C are fruit juices, especially orange juice, and raw foods such as salads made with peppers and spinach.

Healthy Vitamin C

As with beta-carotene, there have been many studies to show that people who eat the most vitamin C have a reduced risk of cancer. According to Professor Gladys Block, a senior nutrition specialist at the National Cancer Institute in America, there is strong evidence for a protective effect of vitamin C against cancers of the oesophagus, larynx and oral cavity. There is also strong, although slightly less consistent, evidence that vitamin C protects against many other cancers including those of the cervix, colon, stomach and pancreas. Even more excitingly, a study by researchers at the University of California has found that those who eat high levels of vitamin C generally live longer and are particularly protected from heart disease. This is possibly because vitamin C works well with its allied antioxidant, vitamin E, which has also been shown to reduce dramatically the risk of heart disease.

Vitamin C Co-stars

Another group of trace-nutrients that are interesting medical researchers are the flavonoids. These are always found together with vitamin C in foods such as citrus fruits and apples, and they may prove to be just as exciting as the ACE vitamins in the future. The flavonoids currently being researched include anthocyanins, flavonols and flavones. These are known to increase the action of vitamin C and help strengthen cell membranes. They may also play a role in preventing heart disease. A study by a team of researchers in the Netherlands published in *The Lancet* in 1993 revealed that the flavonoids in crops such as onions and apples 'may reduce the risk of death from coronary heart disease'. After adjusting their data for other dietary factors, it was shown that it was the specific antioxidant action of the flavonoids that protects against heart disease. Flavonoids can be found in all fruits and vegetables (especially in their skins) which is even more reason why we should be eating more of the ACE super-slimming foods.

Orange-coloured foods are well-known for their antioxidant beta-carotene content, but other colourful fruits and vegetables also have interesting properties. Dark green vegetables contain plenty of cancer-protecting beta-carotene but this is masked by the more dominant green chlorophyll pigment. Chlorophyll itself contains magnesium which is needed for nerve and hormone activity. In addition, dark green vegetables belonging to the *cruciferous* family, such as cabbage, brussel sprouts, kale, broccoli and cauliflower, have been found to protect against cancer. This may be because they contain *indoles*, substances believed to reduce breast-cancer risk. Dark green herbs are also a concentrated source of several interesting antioxidant, including monterpene found in basil and mint. The bright colour of tomatoes, pink grapefruit, strawberries and watermelon comes from the antioxidant lycopene. Another group of colourants are the anthocyanidins, which turn blueberries, blackberries and cherries a deep shade of purple. These compounds have been shown to reduce inflammation in disorders such as arthritis, and may explain why naturopaths recommend cherry and blackberry juice to patients with gout (a common form of arthritis).

Ten Top Sources of Vitamin C
Vitamin C is widely available in many varied fresh fruits and vegetables. Frozen fruits and vegetables also tend to contain good levels of vitamin C.

Food	mg of Vitamin C per 100g (4oz)	Kcals per 100g (4oz)
Guavas	230	26
Blackcurrants	200	28
Green peppers	120	15
Strawberries	77	27
Kale	71	33
Watercress	62	22
Brussels sprouts	60	42
Oranges	54	37
Broccoli	44	33
Tomato purée	38	68

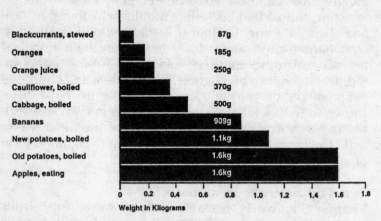

Quantities of foods required to provide 100mg of Vitamin C

Food	Weight
Blackcurrants, stewed	87g
Oranges	185g
Orange juice	250g
Cauliflower, boiled	370g
Cabbage, boiled	500g
Bananas	909g
New potatoes, boiled	1.1kg
Old potatoes, boiled	1.6kg
Apples, eating	1.6kg

Weight in Kilograms

Source: Boots Micronutrients Information Service

Vitamin C Counter

Vitamin C is usually measured in milligrams (mg) or grams (g). 1,000mg is equal to 1g of vitamin C. The recommended daily allowance for adults in Britain is currently a mere 30mg, although the new European recommendation is 60mg and many experts say that even this should be raised to at least 100mg. It is important to eat plenty of vitamin C-rich fruits and vegetables (especially citrus fruits) throughout the day in order to keep our vitamin C levels high. Vitamin C supplements are useful as a back-up to a healthy diet and when we want to boost our intake during times of illness or stress.

Vitamin E

Vitamin E is possibly our most important free-radical fighter because it protects the fats found in all our cells. Vitamin E was first isolated from wheatgerm oil in the 1930s by an American research scientist. It was discovered that the term vitamin E actually covers an entire family of chemical compounds called *tocopherols*, of which d-alpha tocopherol (the natural form of vitamin E) is the most potent. In addition to being a powerful antioxidant and free-radical fighter, vitamin E is essential for maintaining a healthy immune system as it strengthens white blood cells against infection and has a strong link with preventing heart disease. A study by the World Health Organization identified low levels of vitamin E as being the single most important risk factor in death from heart disease – more important even than high cholesterol.

Vitamin E has most recently hit the headlines with the news that it can help to cover our risk of heart disease. A long-term study by Harvard University of over 87,000 women showed that doses of more than 100 IU (international units) of vitamin E a day gave significant protection from heart disease. This protection was *only* seen in those women who were taking a vitamin E supplement. No such results were observed in those who adjusted their diet to include more vitamin E-rich foods. Those who had been taking vitamin E supplements for two or more years had half the risk of heart disease of those who had taken no supplement. This finding is highly significant in terms of long-term better health. It is also of great importance to all slimmers or anyone on any kind of restricted diet who may well be low on vitamin E.

Too little vitamin E in the diet damages good health as it leads to the loss of red blood cells, muscle wastage and eventual sterility. Unfortunately for us, it is not easy to detect when we are lacking in vitamin E as there are few early warning signs. Unlike a vitamin C deficiency, which quickly causes skin bruising, gum disease and (eventually) scurvy, the body gives us few clues that we may be running low on vitamin E. The increase in free radical activity due to environmental factors such as smoking and car-exhaust pollution means that the body has an extra need for vitamin E. Sadly there are few everyday foods that are rich in this important vitamin. This has led many health and nutrition experts to the conclusion that we should take an additional supplement.

Even if you do eat a diet high in foods containing vitamin E, you are only likely to be consuming around 20mg (30 IU) a day. According to Professor Anthony Diplock, head of biochemistry at Guy's Medical School, London, our daily intake should be nearer to 50–80mg (75–120 IU). The many studies in the UK and USA on disease prevention are generally based on much larger amounts of up to 800 IU of vitamin E every day. Vitamin E is a very safe nutrient to supplement. No adverse side-effects have been reported at even 300 times the recommended dose (if only the same were true of synthetic drugs). The best way to achieve a high intake of vitamin E while on a weight-loss diet is to take a daily supplement. Each capsule of vitamin E contains only five calories, yet provides ample antioxidant health protection.

Where to find Vitamin E

Vitamin E is a fat-soluble vitamin. This means that it is found in fatty foods such as vegetable oils, avocados, nuts and seeds. Vitamin E is also found in the protective membrane that surrounds plant cells which is why we find small amounts in vegetables such as asparagus, spinach and wheatgerm. These foods give us useful supplies of vitamin E, but probably do not provide enough of this antioxidant on a daily basis. Vegetable oils are one of the best sources of vitamin E, yet are only used a few drops at a time. Also, many of the foods containing vitamin E, such as oils, nuts and avocados, are very high in fat and are best kept to a minimum while following a weight-loss regime.

Quantities of foods required to provide 75mg of Vitamin E

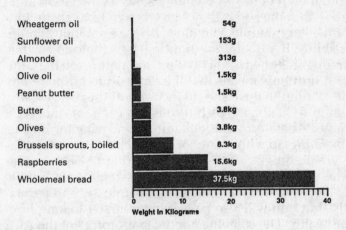

Wheatgerm oil	54g
Sunflower oil	153g
Almonds	313g
Olive oil	1.5kg
Peanut butter	1.5kg
Butter	3.8kg
Olives	3.8kg
Brussels sprouts, boiled	8.3kg
Raspberries	15.6kg
Wholemeal bread	37.5kg

Weight in Kilograms

Source: Boots Micronutrients Information Service

Ten Top Sources of Vitamin E

The best sources of vitamin E are also high in calories, so use sparingly. Those following the weight-loss diet plan should take a 75g (100 IU) Vitamin E supplement.

Food	mg of Vitamin E per 100g (4oz)	Kcals per 100g (4oz)
Wheatgerm oil	136	899
Sunflower oil	49	899
Safflower oil	40	899
Sunflower seeds	38	581
Almonds	24	612
Wheatgerm	22	302
Peanut (groundnut) oil	15	899
Tomato purée	5.3	68
Olive oil	5.1	899
Peanut butter	5	623

ACE Health Allies

Although each of the ACE vitamins has its own individual action within the body, they also work collectively as anti-oxidants. For example, vitamin C helps regenerate vitamin E, enabling it to continue fighting free radicals as they occur in the system. The synergistic nature of the anti-oxidant nutrients means that it is difficult to pinpoint any single vitamin that we should focus on in the diet. Ideally, we should maintain high levels of each of the ACE nutrients – beta-carotene, vitamin C and vitamin E. This means filling up with plenty of ACE-rich fruits, vegetables and whole grains. The idea of eating ACE vitamin-enriched foods gives this weight-loss regime its unique edge: Not only will you lose weight painlessly and perma-nently, but you will also be helping yourself to long-term better health. The combined antioxidant forces of the ACE vitamins will help to prevent many major diseases, in-cluding heart disease and some kinds of cancers. They may even slow down the very ageing process itself, by preventing the free radicals from damaging our cells.

ACE Health Benefits

Beta-carotene
- Powerful cancer preventer
- Speeds the healing process
- Improves eyesight
- Helps prevent heart disease
- Fights infections

Vitamin C
- Protects the heart
- Helps prevent strokes
- Boosts the immune system
- Helps prevent cataracts
- Strengthens blood vessels

- Protects the lungs against pollution
- Reduces the severity of colds and 'flu

Vitamin E
- Reduces the risk of heart disease
- Protects against cancer
- Boosts the immune system
- Protects the lungs against pollution
- Speeds wound healing
- Helps prevent cataracts
- Protects red blood cells
- Helps prevent muscle damage

Clinical Evidence

Over the last few years there have been many hundreds of studies into the extraordinary powers of the ACE vitamins. The British government alone has spent several million pounds researching the very real health benefits offered by these antioxidants. Several of the first major studies into the effects of these vitamins were carried out at the acclaimed Harvard Medical School in Boston, USA. Others have taken place in many other countries around the world, including Britain, where research has been carried out at several centres, including London and Oxford Universities. It is clear that the ACE vitamin-rich foods are more than just a way to get slim and stay slim. They must also become a fundamental part of our diet for better health and a longer life.

Lung Cancer
- One of the longest research projects was a twenty-year study of 4,500 men in Finland. This showed that those with the highest daily intake of beta-carotene, vitamin C and vitamin E had the lowest levels of lung cancer. Even among non-smokers, those with the lowest levels of beta-carotene were *at least twice as likely* to develop lung cancer and die.

Heart Disease and Strokes

- These are Britain's biggest killers of both men and women each year. One of many major research projects at Harvard Medical School, involving 87,000 nurses over eight years, found that those who ate more beta-carotene had 40 percent fewer strokes and 22 percent fewer heart attacks. The same study also found that taking a daily vitamin E supplement reduced the nurses' risk of a heart attack by over 36 percent.

Longevity

- A ten-year study of 11,000 men and women at the University of California found that those who took large amounts of vitamin C every day had a 25-45 percent lower death rate of heart disease and a 10-42 percent reduced mortality from all cancers. A further study of 85,000 people in Finland has shown that daily supplements of the ACE vitamins reduce the risk of developing cancer.

It is never too early or too late to benefit from the health advantages the antioxidants have to offer and clinical evidence continues to mount in favour of the ACE vitamins. The health protection that they offer starts before birth and continues throughout our life into old age. In a study completed in 1993, researchers at the Children's Hospital in Philadelphia discovered that children are less likely to develop brain tumours if their mothers eat plenty of ACE-rich fruits and fruit juices while they are pregnant. Mothers who had eaten ACE-rich foods plus a vitamin C and multi-vitamin supplement gave better protection to their children up to the age of six years old than those who did not. By contrast, a study of 30,000 elderly residents of north-central China, also completed in 1993, showed that those who were given supplements of beta-carotene, vitamin E and selenium (an antioxidant mineral) had a 13 per cent lower risk of death from cancer. Whatever your age, shape or size it is important to include the ACE super-slimming foods in your daily diet – not only for weight-loss, but also for long-term health gain.

5
THE AGES OF ACE EATING

Whatever your age, today is the first day of
the rest of your life

Children

We can learn a lot about the way our bodies like to be
fuelled by watching our own children's eating habits. Kids
often find it difficult to finish large meals, but they all love
to eat snacks. Nutritionists now believe that snacking
throughout the day is OK, provided we are really hungry
and not just bored. This shift in our eating pattern is called
'grazing', and so long as we choose low-fat, ACE vitamin-
rich options, grazing is perfectly fine for a weight-loss
regime. The idea is to cut down on monster-sized meals
with many courses and aim instead for smaller snacks that
will give us a constant energy supply throughout the day.
A study at the University of Toronto found that men who
ate a staggering seventeen snacks per day were actually in
better shape than those who ate three main meals. Not
only were these men leaner, but their cholesterol levels
were lower and they also released more constant levels of
glucose into their bloodstream. In addition, the nibblers

reported that they never felt hungry and could give up sweet and salty snacks more easily than their big-meal counterparts.

Eating much smaller meals more often helps us to avoid over-eating by keeping our blood-sugar levels stable. This means that we don't experience the ravenous hunger-pangs that make us head straight for the biscuit tin. Eating smaller, more frequent meals works well for children who are used to snacking and it is possible for children to enjoy snacks on good, wholesome food. One way is by dividing large meals into smaller portions. For example, if you usually serve a low-fat yogurt after lunch, save it for snack time. You will not be giving yourself or your child any more calories, but you will even out the energy supply from food and avoid a sudden drop. Fruits and vegetables are not only packed with ACE vitamins, they also make good snack-foods. Grapes are ideal for small hands to grasp, for example, and carrot and celery sticks are great to crunch on. The *occasional* refined sugar treat is OK, provided it is just that. Never reward a child with sweets. It is far better to bribe children with exotic fruits, comics, balloons or small toys. This ensures they do not grow up to link sweets and chocolate with good behaviour or associate them with self-esteem.

The fact that children are biologically programmed to eat little and often should be encouraged. The danger lies in eating junk food snacks. Unfortunately, the food industry promotes the unhealthiest types of snacks and targets them specifically at our children. Today, British schoolchildren eat more sweets, chocolate and high-fat savoury snacks than in any other European country! More than 6,000 million small bags of crisps are sold in Britain each year – mostly to children. These high-fat, high-salt snacks are also often combined with a chocolate snack, which pushes a child's daily fat consumption way over the safe limit. Not surprisingly, nearly half of all five-year-olds suffer from tooth decay. This visible effect of their poor diets would be even more apparent were it not for the protective effect of fluoride in our toothpaste and tap water.

Of the 140 children's foods launched in 1992, more than half were sugared chocolate, soft drinks and high-fat snack foods. In the same year, the food industry spent over £100 million advertising confectionery alone. Sugar companies also fund the Sugar Bureau, which promotes 'education' packs and project material in schools, encouraging the use of sugar in cooking and processed foods. These project packs are fun and highly visual, without a fat person or tooth filling in sight. The highly dubious decision to target children with unhealthy foods is due to the very real 'pester-power' that children exert over their parents' shopping. The National Food Alliance pressure group estimates that 'pester power' is worth at least £1.25 billion a year to the food industry. With two small children myself, I know only too well just how difficult it is *not* to give in to a screaming toddler throwing a tantrum in the supermarket. However hard it is to cut back on the fatty, sugary foods, you owe it to your child's health and well-being to try.

Given the choice, children tend to eat a lot of sugary foods and this is very often at the expense of more nutritious alternatives. The average diet of the under 12s has been found to be high in fat and sugar and low in vital vitamins and body-building minerals. One study by Professor Rugg-Gunn at Newcastle University found that chips and crisps were the largest source of energy for an average group of eleven-year-olds. Professor Rugg-Gunn also found that their vitamin A and iron levels were low compared to government regulations. In 1990, an additional study revealed that every week the average British eleven-year-old consumed the following: seven bars of chocolate or other sweets, seven biscuits, six cans of soft drinks and four packets of crisps. Few chose to eat any fruit or vegetables at all – so where are their vitamins and body-building minerals coming from?

The food industry will not admit to the damage that these unhealthy foods can cause. Charts produced by SNACMA (the Snack Nut and Crisp Manufacturers' Association) to show the nutrient content of crisps do not even mention the word 'fat'. Their extraordinarily high fat content is misrepresented as 'vegetable' content – presumably because the fat comes from vegetable oils. Lower-fat crisps are even labelled with the words 'can help you lose weight only when part of a calorie controlled diet'. However, as even 'lower-fat' crisps contain more fat than chocolate digestive biscuits it would be more accurate to state that they are of no earthly use at all. You can see from just these two examples alone how difficult it is to make informed choices about the right foods for successful slimming. When in doubt, read the label to discover a snack's fat content. If this is not listed, contact the manufacturer.

Fat Snacks	
Snack	**fat per 100g**
dry roasted peanuts (average)	49g
KP ready salted peanuts	39g
Hedgehog lightly sea salted crisps	39g
Smiths ready salted crisps	38g
Golden Wonder ready salted crisps	35g
milk chocolate (average)	30g
KP lower fat lightly salted crisps	28g
milk chocolate digestives (average)	20g

If weight-gain and ill-health is to be avoided in later life it is imperative to start children on the right track from infancy. It is much more difficult (though not impossible) to retrain a sweet tooth once it has taken hold. Babies have a natural preference for sweet foods such as soft foods, but this is no excuse to skimp on nutrition and pile on the calories. Eating patterns are set in childhood and studies show that a baby's taste buds can easily cope with fresh, wholesome foods. One of the most important times for infant feeding seems to be around six to eighteen months, when they will develop a liking for many different fruits and vegetables if given the chance. Professor Jeffrey Blumberg, Associate Director of the Human Nutrition Research

Center in Boston, USA insists that healthy eating should start young. He points out that children as young as eight years old have been found to have the fatty streaks in their arteries that lead to heart disease. It is these children who are especially at risk from being significantly overweight and low in energy in later life. So don't choose the easy option. Boycott the advertisers' colourful packaging, snazzy labels and fancy monster shapes. Your child's future health and well-being is at stake.

Your Kids Need ACE-eating Habits
- Children need nutritious diets to develop and grow
- Life-long eating habits begin in childhood
- Lack of ACE vitamins leads to ill-health in later life
- Tooth decay is one of the most common childhood ailments
- Obese children have high blood pressure and increased cholesterol levels
- Good health, vitality and lifelong well-being are the best gifts you can give your children.

Teenagers

The British trend for unhealthy eating increases as children get older. The results of a nationwide survey of ten- to fifteen-year-olds commissioned by Channel Four television in 1993 are disturbing. More than 50 percent *never* eat fruit and vegetables, 40 percent eat chips *every day*, and 22 percent of *all* teenage girls go without breakfast. If over-eating the wrong types of fattening foods is the main problem during childhood, under-eating can be a more common problem in adolescence. Most teenage girls adopt some form of restricted eating regime, whether it is a fad-diet, a longer term slimming plan or simply becoming a vegetarian. The problem is that dieting during adolescence can seriously damage health. Any kind of restricted eating inevitably restricts the amounts of nutrients available in the diet. Unfortunately, adolescence is one of the key times when we need the best nutrition possible for healthy physical development.

The worry of weight-loss is also a common trigger for many serious eating disorders. A survey conducted by the British Psychological Society revealed that girls as young as nine years old are dieting. Teenage girls are most at risk from frequent dieting and it is important not to under-estimate the overwhelming impact of our diet-culture on adolescents. As a teenager I was not overweight, yet I counted calories, followed the latest fad diets and ago-nized over every mouthful. In fact, I was shocked to real-ize while writing this book that it has taken almost two decades for me to feel relaxed about eating. Many others are not so fortunate. Anorexia nervosa is an emotional dis-order characterized by a fear of becoming fat and a pre-occupation with food. It has become increasingly common amongst teenage girls (it is rare in males and adult women). Yet we do need some body fat to survive. If a girl's body fat falls below 18 percent of her total weight, her periods will stop and she may even become infertile. Anorexia nervosa involves a total withdrawal from eating, which also dramatically damages the body's metabolism and can ultimately end in death.

Bulimia is another serious eating disorder that focuses on an unhealthy obsession with food. The typical binge and purge cycle of bulimics greatly undermines their health, the persistent vomiting rots their teeth and often continues as an obsessive illness throughout their life. Un-fortunately, these eating disorders most commonly strike during adolescence at the very time when the body is try-ing to develop and grow. We now know that most of our calcium deposits are laid down during our teenage years and this is an important factor in creating bone strength. Unless we lay down the solid foundations of a healthy body during adolescence, we are unlikely to develop in a healthy way. This is especially important for teenage girls, who may become most at risk from osteoporosis (brittle bones) if they make it to middle age.

The best way to overcome teenage 'puppy fat', regulate

weight fluctuations and build the strongest body possible for the future is to adopt the principles of ACE-eating. Instead of seeing meal-times as a battle zone, *Weight-Loss for Life* encourages teenagers to make friends with food and to recognize it as the ultimate for a fit, strong and active body. Learning to cook healthy, ACE vitamin-rich meals is also a top priority. As a nation, we seem to be losing our ability to prepare even the simplest meals. A 1993 MORI poll of seven- to fifteen-year-olds discovered that while 93 percent knew how to play video games, only 38 percent could cook a basic jacket potato in the oven. Asked what dishes they could make, barely half said they could boil an egg and only 67 percent could put together a salad. Fortunately, the principles of ACE-eating for weight-loss are reassuringly simple and all the recipes in this book are fuss-free. Regardless of what you like to cook, one of the best moves you can make as a parent is to teach your children the ACE cooking skills that will last them a lifetime.

ACE Adolescence

- Encourage your teenager to cook. Buy an exotic cookery book, delegate cooking the Sunday lunch, keep a scrapbook of magazine recipes – anything to fuel their interest.
- Teenagers eat more savoury snacks and takeaway foods such as meat pies, burgers and kebabs than any other population group. Introduce them to the low-fat alternatives on pages 30, 33 and 36.
- Fizzy-drinks are bad news for growing bodies as they are high in phosphates which block the absorption of calcium. Teenagers should switch to ACE vitamin-rich fruit juices for the sake of their teeth and bones.
- Watch out for food fads, including crash diets and vegetarianism. There is nothing wrong with healthy, low-fat eating or well-balanced vegetarian meals. However, any kind of restricted eating habit needs monitoring to make sure young people get their full share of nutrients for a healthy future.

Adults

By the time we reach adulthood most of our eating patterns have been firmly established. We know what foods we like and how we like them cooked. The older we are, the more set in our ways we become. Any attempt to revolutionize adult eating habits overnight is doomed to failure. This book is about achieving weight-loss *for life*. It does not, therefore, urge you to throw out all the food in your freezer and restock the cupboards with alfalfa sprouts and mung beans. What it does suggest is that you think rationally about the way you choose, prepare, stock and cook food for yourself and members of your family. Small differences and gradual changes in eating patterns will make a dramatic difference to both your waistline and your well-being.

It is estimated that about 80 percent of all British food is processed – more than in almost any other country in the world. While some of these foods are low in fat and high in fibre, the majority are not. The recipes that you will find in the twenty-eight-day *Weight-Loss for Life* eating plan are based on large quantities of complex carbohydrates (rice, beans, pasta, potatoes etc.) and plenty of the ACE vitamin-rich fruits and vegetables. Although the regime is not strictly vegetarian it does not include very much animal produce. The reason for this is that animal produce, such as meat and cheese, contains high levels of saturated fats and we should keep these to a minimum. However, you will find several fish and seafood recipes as these contain mono- and polyunsaturated fats, as well as useful amounts of protein. Those who are vegetarian will find most of the recipes are suitable for them. There are also plenty of vegetarian alternatives for those who don't eat chicken or fish.

The Meat-eating Option
These days there is no risk of running low on protein by not eating as there are plenty of high-protein alternatives.

Good sources of protein include fish, eggs, dairy produce, nuts, seeds, rice and beans. However, meat does contain valuable amounts of iron and this mineral is especially important for women. Iron deficiency is worryingly common in women, especially those who have heavy periods as they lose a significant amount of their iron supplies this way every month. Red meat is by far our best source of absorbable iron and the occasional portion three or four times a month is a good option for the demi-vegetarian. If you do eat meat you should choose it carefully. Free-range and organically reared meat is not only far more humane, it is also better for your health. Animals that are allowed to run free have more lean tissue and less fat than those reared on factory farms. As an example, the fat content of a pig is around 30 percent compared to just 1–2 percent from a free-ranging hog. Factory farmed animals are also routinely fed antibiotics and synthetic growth hormones and it is the modern unnatural feeding practices that have resulted in the rise of BSE 'mad cow' disease. Although free-range meat costs more it is well worth the extra money. Vegetarian or not, no one needs to eat the amounts of meat that justify barbaric modern farming processes.

Meal Times
Another factor that features in weight-loss is the time of day when we eat our meals. Back in the 1940s Adele Davis, one of the founder members of the healthy eating revolution, recommended that we should 'eat like a king at breakfast, a prince at lunchtime and a pauper in the evening'. Her point was that our bodies need refuelling for the rigours of the day ahead in the morning. By lunchtime we need a little more to keep us going, but in the evening we should not overload our digestive systems just before going to bed. Unfortunately, our eating habits are more likely to be reversed, with many of us skipping breakfast, having just a sandwich for lunch and then a large dinner late in the evening.
- Daily calories – burnt as fuel
- Evening calories – stored as fat

The problem with eating a big meal in the evening is that we have no time to use the fuel from our food in the form of energy. If we eat just before going to bed the body shuts down and goes to sleep, stashing away those extra calories in our hips and thighs. This problem is solved by eating earlier and making supper a smaller meal. Try bringing the time supper is served forward by half an hour at a time – just make sure you don't end up eating tea as well as a late-night snack! As a last resort, the body finds it easier to convert carbohydrate foods into energy than fatty foods. So if you are planning to eat late one evening, choose starchy foods such as pasta, baked potatoes, beans, rice and pulses which the body will more easily burn off than fats, such as red meat and cheese.

Snack Attack

The snacks we choose have the power to make or break your *Weight-Loss for Life* regime. It is so easy to slip into the habit of eating a chocolate bar every day or dipping into the biscuit barrel with every coffee break. The best way to switch on to healthier snacks is to identify exactly *when* you get the urge to reach for something sweet. Mid-morning snack attacks frequently hit us when our blood-sugar levels dip. This occurs when we have not eaten enough of the complex carbohydrates for breakfast. Eating a large ACE vitamin-rich breakfast will curb these artificial hunger pangs and you will find details of the delicious Big ACE Breakfast on page 94.

We often find ourselves reaching for a snack out of habit or boredom. Think of what triggers your motivation. Are you really hungry – or just fed up? It may be that you always have something sweet with a cup of tea or you might always dip into a bag of crisps when you watch a video. The key is to identify these fattening habits so that you can take evasive action. Changing your habits will remove the psychological association with certain foods. The key to successful snacking is to have plenty of healthy options in the house or at work. The so-called 'diet' chocolate bars and biscuits don't work for weight-loss in the long-term because they ignore our need to develop a taste for healthier options. It is extraordinary that a new 'low calorie' Mars bar is now available in the United States, which contains 25 percent fewer calories. Mars have plans to launch lower-calorie chocolates made with one of the new synthetic fats, worldwide. But synthetic, highly processed junk foods are not the answer for life-long health and permanent weight-loss. It is the ACE vitamin-rich foods that give us the nutrients and energy for a lighter, leaner shape.

- Drink herb teas instead of regular tea and replace biscuits with a bunch of grapes or an apple.
- Popcorn is a great low-calorie snack, provided you eat it plain without butter, oil or sugar. Keep a bag of popping corn in the kitchen cupboard ready for when you fancy something crunchy to snack on.
- If you tend to raid the fridge in search of a late-night snack, make sure you have a bag of chopped carrot and celery sticks ready for munching.
- If biscuits are your weakness stock the tin with rice cakes instead. They have far fewer calories but make a satisfying snack.
- If you absolutely must have some chocolate, buy a small bar of very dark, plain chocolate which contains less sugar than milk varieties. Limit yourself to one a week.
- Seedless grapes contain plenty of natural fruit sugars and will satisfy the sweetest tooth.
- Alcohol weakens the resolve. If you can't have a glass of wine without a bowl of peanuts drink mineral water or fruit juice instead.
- You are allowed the occasional lapse! After all, to err is human, to forgive is divine. You will have renewed motivation if you learn to love and respect your body.

The Elderly

It is a sad fact of life that as we grow older we tend to grow fatter. Our average Body Mass Index (BMI), a measurement used by health professionals to assess obesity, tends to be higher in the older age groups. This because we are more likely to eat sweet and fatty foods, such as butter, cream, milk puddings and confectionery. The 1990 Dietary and Nutritional Survey of British Adults found that 75 percent of all elderly adults regularly eat biscuits and cakes as against just 30 percent regularly eating pasta and rice. Switching on to healthy ACE eating in our early years makes it easier to beat bad habits before they take hold. However, it is never too late to enjoy the very real benefits that come with *Weight-Loss for Life*.

Osteoporosis

The bone disease known as osteoporosis is a common part of the ageing process that affects about one-third of all women over the age of 65. As osteoporosis progresses our bones become thinner and weaker, making them more likely to break or fracture. Eating plenty of calcium and taking regular exercise will help prevent loss of bone mass due to age. This is one reason why this book pays extra attention to both calcium-rich foods and the importance of exercise. Before the menopause, women need approximately 800–100mg of calcium a day. After the menopause, women may need as much as 1200mg of calcium daily.

Dairy products are an obvious source of calcium but they can also be high in saturated fat. The Milk Marketing Board has done such a good job in educating us about our needs for calcium that we often forget that there are many other excellent sources of calcium apart from dairy foods. For example, green leafy vegetables such as broccoli and Swiss chard are good sources of calcium, as are tinned salmon and sardines (eaten with their bones). Calcium is such an important part of our daily diet that you will find plenty of calcium-rich recipes with these ingredients later in this book. The *Weight-Loss for Life* twenty-eight-day eating plan also includes a daily Frothy Yogurt Shake, which contains around 200mg of bone-building calcium, in each glass. Those who don't drink cow's milk or eat dairy foods can replace the skimmed milk in this with calcium-enriched soya milk.

In addition to calcium, there is no getting away from the fact that regular exercise is also especially important for mature women. Like muscles, our bones become stronger with use. This is why weight-bearing exercises such as walking or jogging are so useful in later life to strengthen and thicken our bones. A study carried out at Nottingham University showed that regular, daily jumping for a year increased the density of hip bones in pre-menopausal women by a substantial 3 percent. In this study, the women made fifty jumps a day, which takes no longer than cleaning your teeth. The impact of jumping up and down on the ground seems to be enough to stimulate healthy bone formation.

ACE Old Age

One side-effect of inactivity in old age is that the elderly find themselves prone to weight-gain as they slow down. To compensate for this, more emphasis should be placed on healthy ACE-eating. You are never too old to benefit from the many advantages of adopting a healthier eating regime. Indeed, many of the very disorders that affect the elderly, such as cataracts, arthritis and heart disease can be prevented by the unique antioxidant ACE vitamins in food. The British government has finally recognized that more needs to be done to encourage healthy eating amongst the elderly. In 1992, a report by the Committee of Medical Aspects of Food Policy (COMA) entitled *The Nutrition of Elderly People* made no less than forty-two recommendations for improving eating habits. This was the first in-depth report for more than twenty years and uncovered some disturbing statistics.

The COMA report expressed concern that the elderly were simply not receiving sufficient nutrients in their food to prevent many diseases. It was noted that many elderly people are being admitted to hospital suffering from poor nutrition and that this is not being detected early enough. It was recommended that all elderly people should be advised to eat much more fibre, fruit, vegetables and vitamins A, C and D. They should also dramatically decrease their intake of fat and salt. These guidelines exactly follow the *Weight-Loss for Life* healthy eating principles. If the elderley make the simple switch to ACE-eating, they will not only find that they lose excess pounds, but that they also feel fitter, stronger and are better protected against many of the degenerative and life-threatening diseases.

There have been several studies showing that the elderly benefit from taking vitamin and mineral supplements. Researchers in Newfoundland examined the effects of daily doses of vitamins on the health of men and women over the age of sixty-five. In a controlled trial for one year ninety-six volunteers given antioxidant ACE vitamins had their immune system boosted (shown by laboratory tests) and had far fewer days of illness (seven days of sickness as against twenty-three). The antioxidant vitamins also have many extra health benefits that are increasingly important in later life. For example, studies have highlighted the importance of the ACE vitamins in helping to prevent many degenerative disorders such as cataracts and they may even play a role in preventing arthritis. As we have seen in the previous chapter, the ACE antioxidant nutrients are fundamental in helping to prevent many of the diseases that are common in later life. Increasing your intake of these vitamin-rich foods will not only improve your figure, but will also go a long way in effective, preventative medical care.

ACE-Eating in Old Age

- Take it slowly! Your weight-loss will not happen overnight. It may have taken several decades for the pounds to pile on, so they will not disappear in a few weeks. Long-term goals are more achievable.
- Are you too set in your ways when it comes to food? Try new varieties of vegetables an the newer exotic fruits now available. Remember that the more colourful they are, the more ACE vitamins they contain.
- Change your eating habits – if you can't pass a bakery

without buying a sticky bun then change your route! If you always buy sweets when you pick up your pension ask someone else to do it for you. If you have always had second helpings, practise saying No.

- If you are cooking meals for just one person, remember that frozen vegetables have good levels of the ACE vitamins and are more convenient for single portions.
- Involve your family. If you make the switch to healthier eating let the others know so that they won't sabotage your plans by bringing fattening gifts or cooking fat-filled meals.

6
ACE WEIGHT-LOSS – LET'S GO!

Never put off until tomorrow what you can
do today

Over the next few pages you will find the twenty-eight-day starter slimming plan that sets you on your own personal weight-loss for life. This four-week eating plan has been carefully devised to give you one complete month of delicious recipes. Each recipe and menu idea has been carefully put together to maximize vitamin values while minimizing the fat and calorie content. Every day you will be able to choose a tasty option for breakfast, lunch and supper – as well as mid-morning and tea-time snacks and special treats. The key to successful slimming is to eat little and often, choosing ACE vitamin-rich foods including plenty of whole grins, fresh fruits and vegetables. This first month of the *Weight-Loss for Life* eating plan is guaranteed to mobilize fat cells and shift surplus pounds while boosting your metabolism and energy levels. The twenty-eight-day eating plan sets you well on the way to achieving your target figure and for successful, life-long weight maintenance.

Breakfast First

Breakfast is the most important meal of the day for all of us who want to lose weight. The word breakfast literally means 'breaking the fast' and it is vital that we do not skip this vital part of the day. Having breakfast boosts our blood sugar levels and fuels the body for the day ahead. Nutritional studies in both Britain and the United States show that skipping breakfast is a false economy as our body will under-perform for the rest of the day. This is especially true for children who leave home with an empty stomach. By mid-morning their behaviour and ability in the classroom is significantly worse than that of those who have eaten a good breakfast.

So what is the best breakfast? Unfortunately the traditional British fare of fried bread, bacon, sausages and fried eggs is so full of fat that it slides right off the plate and into our hungry fat cells. The very occasional cooked breakfast is fine – but forget the fried bread, make sure the bacon is grilled, add plenty of tomatoes and a single poached egg to reduce the fat content by more than half. Sausages are just too stuffed with fat, rusk, preservatives and leftover bits of gristle to be taken seriously as a form of food. Substitute with a lean lamp chop, or better still, a grilled kipper. However, for our day-to-day breakfasts we should be switching to cereals and toast. Not only are these lower in fat, they also contain the important complex carbohydrates that give us a wonderfully steady energy supply for the day ahead.

Cereal Choice

Many processed cereals are sold with a 'healthy' tag, but just how healthy are they? Surprisingly, some are not as good for us as their makers would have us believe. For example, granola-style mueslis are often high in fat and can contain 45 percent sugar! Even good old All Bran is 15 percent sugar (and that's before you add an extra spoonful of the white stuff). Kellog's Special K is promoted as the slimmer's cereal, yet it contains 57 times more sugar than puffed wheat. And although some cereals such as Frosties, Coco Pops and Smacks may declare themselves to be 'low in fat' they conveniently fail to mention that they are also very high in sugar (Smacks is a whopping 50 percent sugar).

Breakfast Cereal Chart
(measurement in grams per 100g)

Cereal	Total Fats	Total Sugars	Kcal
All Bran	2.5	19	261
Bran Flakes	1.6	18.7	318
Coco Pops	0.9	38.2	384
Oat Bran Flakes	2.4	16.8	357
Corn Flakes	0.5	8.2	360
Crunchy Nut Corn Flakes	3.8	36.3	398
Frosties	0.4	41.9	377
Muesli (average)	5.2	26.2	363
Muesli (no added sugar)	7.4	15.7	366
Porridge (made with water)	1.0	Almost Nil	49
Porridge (made with full-fat milk)	4.7	4.7	116
Puffed Wheat	1.0	0.3	321
Ready Brek (plain)	6.6	1.7	373
Rice Kispies	0.8	10.6	369
Ricicles	0.5	41.9	381
Shredded Wheat	2.2	0.8	325
Shreddies	1.1	10.2	331
Smacks	1.5	50.0	386
Special K	0.9	17.2	377
Start	1.4	29.1	355
Sugar Puffs	0.6	56.5	324
Weetabix	2.0	5.2	352
Weetos	1.9	33.2	372

Small differences in taste can make a big change to your waistline – Crunchy Nut Cornflakes have over seven times more fat and almost five times as much sugar as ordinary cornflakes. Chosen carefully, cereals can be the very best start to the day. All health food shops offer a good choice of low-fat, sugar-free cereals, otherwise supermarkets stock good choices, such as porridge oats, Puffed Wheat, Shredded Wheat and Weetabix. The trick is not to ruin the goodness by adding extra sugar. A bowl of sugar-free cereal with semi-skimmed milk is quick, easy and convenient. It is also a great source of fibre, carbohydrate for fuel and calcium for strong teeth and bones.

The Big ACE Breakfast

The Big ACE Breakfast is not to be missed! While following the *Weight-Loss for Life* diet plan, choose from the following selection each and every morning: Bowl of unsweetened cereal with semi-skimmed or skimmed milk. Top with slices of fresh, seasonal fruit, such as apple, pear or strawberries.
or ACE Wake-Up Shake (recipe on page 133)
or ACE Compôte (recipe on page 134)
or Bircher Muesli (recipe on page 135)
Followed by: one slice of wholemeal bread *or* four low-salt crispbreads *or* 4 low-salt rice cakes, spread with one tsp butter *or* low fat spread *or* one tsp smooth sugar-free peanut butter
Served with: one small glass of fresh juice, either apple, orange, tomato *or* carrot juice (or a combination).

ACE Breakfast Tips

Here are some ideas that the entire family can follow to boost their breakfast each morning:
● Drink an extra glass of fresh fruit juice every morning before breakfast. The best choices are orange, apple,

cranberry, carrot and tomato.

- Use fresh bread which is moist enough not to need butter – you will find a delicious recipe for Quick-Cook Wholemeal Bread on page 136.
- Switch to low-fat diet spreads, or use low-sugar fruit spreads on bread and toast instead of butter.
- Cereals are a low-fat option. Choose sugar-free versions that are also high in fibre (see chart on page 93)
- Add fresh or dried fruit to cereal to boost its ACE vitamin content.
- Switch to skimmed or semi-skimmed milk and save fat grams.

Snacks

Eating a generous breakfast will stabilize blood-sugar levels for the morning and means we are less likely to feel hungry. However, regular snackers will find it useful to snack on healthy, low-calorie foods during the day to ward off hunger pangs. While following the unique ACE vitamin-rich eating plan, you will have plenty of opportunity to snack on healthy foods. Each morning, you are allowed the choice of an ACE juice cocktail or a fresh fruit snack. Fresh fruit and fruit juices are the best choices for a mid-morning snack as they are low in calories, rich in energy-giving vitamins and with a little extra fibre to fill the stomach.

Fresh fruit and fruit juices are also packed with enzymes that improve the digestion. These enzymes are only found in fresh juices as they are easily destroyed by the heat treatment, including pasteurization, that many cartoned juices are subjected to. In an ideal world, fresh fruit juices should come straight from the fruit. If this is not possible, buy freshly squeezed juices from the chill cabinet. If you want to squeeze your own, citrus fruits are the easiest to juice, either with an electric orange squeezer or by hand. Other fruit juices can be extracted with a centrifugal juice extractor, which is an electric processor that grinds fruits and vegetables against a whirring sieve to separate the juice from the fibrous part of the plant. These are about the same price as a food processor and are an excellent investment for any health-conscious cook. Not only can you squeeze the juice from fruits such as apple, peach and pear, but you can also add a few basil leaves or chopped celery stems to turn a glass of tomato juice into an exotic fresh vegetable cocktail.

Mid-Morning Snacks

You are allowed 250ml (8fl oz) of the following fruit juices, or try these delicious cocktail combinations. Each ACE Juice Cocktail should measure 250ml (8 fl oz), which is roughly equivalent to a medium-sized tumbler.

Plain Juices
- Apple
- Orange
- Carrot
- Tomato
- Grapefruit

ACE Juice Cocktails
- one part apple, one part orange, dash of grapefruit
- one part orange, one part apple, one part carrot
- one part pear, one part apricot, one part apple
- one part cranberry, one part apple, pinch of cinnamon
- one part tomato, one part apple, dash of celery
- one part carrot, one part watercress, dash of lemon
- one part tomato, one part spinach, dash of fresh basil
- one part pear, one part apple, one part mango

ACE Fruit Snacks
As an alternative to the ACE Juice Cocktails, you may choose one of the options from the following list of mid-morning fruit snacks
- one apple, pear, orange or banana

- one nectarine, one peach, two fresh or dried apricots
- small bunch of grapes
- one-sixth cantaloupe or water melon
- 50g (2oz) raisins, prunes, dates, or dried apple rings
- 2 fresh or dried figs
- 2 mandarins or clementines
- half fresh papaya or mango

ACE Lunch-Box Selection

This section has been included for all those who take a packed lunch to school or work. When choosing your lunchtime option from the twenty-eight-day meal planner, you may either have the main lunch choice or choose from the lunch-box selection below:

- 100g (4oz) lean meat, fish, seafood *or* low-fat cottage cheese, or ½ small avocado
- with two thin slices of wholemeal bread, *or* eight crispbreads *or* eight low-salt rice cakes, with 2tsp butter or low-fat spread
- with unlimited amounts of tomatoes, spring onions, celery, lettuce, alfalfa sprouts, cucumber, radishes, watercress, carrots and beetroot.

Tea-Time Snacks

We all know that feeling we get around tea-time when our stomach tells our brain that it has finished digesting lunch and can't wait until supper before needing some more sustenance. The ACE *Weight-Loss for Life* eating plan actually allows you to snack – provided it is on healthy ACE vitamin-rich foods. By tea-time we often fancy something sweet and a little bit different. We tend to get sugar cravings at around this time of day as our blood-sugar levels begin to dip two to three hours after lunch. This is the time to try one of the fabulous Frothy Yogurt Shakes (recipe on page 98). Made with low-fat yogurt, these are an excellent choice for slimmers as they are filling and nutritious, without being fattening. Yogurt is also an excellent source of calcium, a mineral which builds strong bones, and it is especially important for women to maintain high levels of calcium to reduce the risk of osteoporosis in later life. Even in old age, eating plenty of calcium in the diet helps to boost bone density and significantly reduces the risk of stress fractures and curvature of the spine (the dreaded dowager's hump).

For those who don't fancy a yogurt drink, try a small pot of low-fat yogurt instead. There are scores of varieties to choose from and they are easy to take into work or add to a lunch box. When choosing a low-fat yogurt, look at the label to make sure that it contains more fruit than sugar (fruit should come first on the added ingredients panel). Many low-fat yogurts are sweetened with artificial sweeteners and these are fine for those following the weight-loss plan. In some supermarkets you can even find 'very low-fat' varieties of yogurt and these have the lowest fat and calorie content of all. If you want to add your own flavourings, buy a large pot of plain, low-fat yogurt and add unsweetened fruit purées (jars of unsweetened baby food fruit purées are ideal), a scant teaspoonful of maple syrup or a sprinkling of chopped nuts. For those who make their own yogurts from scratch, use skimmed milk to reduce the fat content and stir in the flavourings once the yogurt has set.

Frothy Yogurt Shakes

Serves one

50g (2oz) low-fat, plain yogurt
150ml (¼ pint) skimmed milk
1 tbsp fresh fruit flavourings, e.g. mashed banana, strawberries, redcurrants, apple purée, chopped apricots, ground almonds or sliced mango.

Mix the yogurt with the skimmed milk in a blender or whisk together in a bowl. Add the fruit flavouring and mix until frothy. Pour into a tall tumbler and serve immediately. Try experimenting with a combination of flavours. Some of the most successful combinations include apricot and banana, apple and strawberry and banana with almonds.

ACE Drinking

Alcohol is loaded with calories so needs to be drunk with caution while you are following the weight-loss plan. Just one pint of beer contains 180 calories, so you can see how easy it is to pile on the pounds by drinking alcohol. Obviously, drinking to excess also damages your liver. This is because the liver is like a car with only one gear which always goes at the same rate. Overloading the liver with excessive drinking causes chronic damage as the liver is unable to cope with the extra quantity of alcohol. Although a small amount of 'social' drinking is unlikely to cause the liver too many problems, it will interfere with nutrient absorption. Alcohol depletes vitamin A, the B complex vitamins, vitamin C, magnesium, and zinc. In addition, drinking alcohol also encourages the body to absorb lead and aluminium. While this is not serious in the short-term, you should be especially aware of eating vitamin-rich foods while drinking alcohol.

Your ACE Allowance

While following the *Weight-Loss for Life* eating plan you are allowed to drink 3–4 small glass of wine (or their equivalent) each week. It is best to spread this throughout the week and not drink your allowance in one evening. Once you have completed the twenty-eight-day initial weight-loss regime, you should limit your alcohol intake to sensible levels. The Health Education Authority advises that women should drink no more than fourteen units and men no more than twenty-one units, spread throughout a week. Women have a lower allowance than men because of the differing water content in their bodies.

Beer, lager and cider	Calories	Units of Alcohol
Half pint (284ml, 10fl oz) of:		
Bitter	90	1
Brown ale	80	1
Strong ale or lager	85	2
Low-alcohol lager	60	0.25
Dry cider	95	1
Sweet cider	110	1
Strong cider	100	2

Wine	Calories	Units of Alcohol
Average small glass (113ml, 4fl oz) of:		
Dry white wine	75	1
Rosé	85	1
Sweet white wine	85	1
Champagne	70	1

Fortified Wine	Calories	Units of Alcohol
1 pub measure (50ml, ⅓ gill) of:		
Dry sherry or similar	55	1
Medium sherry	60	1
Cream sherry	70	1

Spirits	Calories	Units of Alcohol
1 single measure (25ml, ⅙ gill) of:		
brandy, whisky, gin, rum or vodka	50	1

N.B. Northern Ireland and some parts of Scotland serve larger single measures (¼ gill) which are proportionately higher in calories and count as 1½ units each.

In men, between 55 and 65 percent of the body weight is made up of water. In women, between 45 and 55 percent is water. Alcohol is distributed throughout the body fluids, so in men it is more 'diluted' than in women. In addition, a woman's liver is smaller and more likely to suffer damage than a man's.

What's in a Drink?

Keep track of what and how much you drink with the chart on page 103. If you're concerned about your drinking, switch to low-alcohol lagers, drink de-alcoholized wine or make spritzers with white wine and sparkling mineral water. Low-calorie mixers such as tonic and bitter lemon are also good options, or you could try one of the ACE low-alcohol cocktail recipes on page 199-200.

A Healthy Approach

Some studies have found a protective link between a moderate intake of alcohol (one to two units a day) and heart disease – so should we be drinking more alcohol? Unfortunately, the answer is no, as there are many different reasons why alcohol may *appear* to be good for the heart. Firstly, we tend to drink alcohol when we sit down with friends and it could be this social destressing factor that lowers our risk of coronary heart disease, not the alcohol itself. Also, ex-problem drinkers who have become teetotal fall into the non-drinking section when tested and will distort that group's statistics with their lingering health problems.

In several studies, red wine has been shown to help protect the arteries by preventing the oxidation of LDL (the 'bad' form of cholesterol). Red wine has an effect because it contains antioxidant from the grape skins that are left in contact with the wine during its vinification process. However, as alcohol depletes several other nutrients in the body (notably the B complex vitamins) it can hardly be called a nutritious drink. If you are after antioxidant action from grape skins you are far better off eating a bunch of grapes!

Drink to Your Health

Another problem with drinking alcohol is that it reduces the amount of water within the system. This is because alcohol blocks the action of an anti-diuretic hormone, so the more you drink, the more dehydrated you become. The way to drink healthily is to match each alcoholic drink with a large glass of water. This ensures that fluid is put back into the system to replace the water lost by drinking alcohol. Water is especially important for good health and weight-loss. It is important not to forget to drink plenty of water on a daily basis. Water is a natural detoxifier, helping to sloosh out the build-up of toxins inside the system by binding them with the fibre from our ACE fruits and vegetables.

Drinking water half an hour before a meal also gives you a temporary sense of fullness and helps prevent hunger pangs. The best time to drink water is half an hour before or after a meal. This allows time for food to be efficiently digested by the concentrated acids in the stomach. Try to drink water throughout the day instead of one or two very large glassfuls at one go. Remember – if you feel thirsty, your body probably dehydrated twenty minutes ago. Tap water contains nitrates, chlorine, aluminium and other substances, so it is worth investing in a filter jug, and never use water from the hot tap as it is constantly re-heated which affects its mineral content. It helps to keep a large bottle of low-sodium (salt) mineral water on your desk or in the kitchen and aim to finish it every day.

Drinking Check List

How many units in the last week?

Day	How much?	When/Where/ Who with?	Calories	Units
Monday				
Tuesday				
Wednesday				
Thursday				
Friday				
Saturday				
Sunday				
Totals for the week:				

The Four-Week *Weight-Loss for Life* Menu Plan

The following plan lists all the recipe suggestions you will need for the month ahead. You may switch the lunch option with the supper choice if this is more convenient for you. However, it is important to eat the ACE-rich fresh fruit snacks every day and to make sure you choose at least one carbohydrate-based meal a day. You will find plenty of the dishes include rice, bread, pulses or potatoes which will fill you up with energy-giving complex carbohydrates. While following the twenty-eight-day eating plan, you should drink six to eight glasses of water a day. This will help to create the feeling of fullness. Try not to drink any liquids half an hour before or after a meal, as this dilutes the stomach juices that are involved with the process of digestion. You may also drink up to four small glasses of wine, beer or cider each week while following the plan.

Four-week menu plan

WEEK 1	Breakfast	Mid-morning snack	Lunch	Tea-time snack	Supper
Monday	ACE breakfast choice (page 94)	ACE juice cocktail or ACE fruit snack (page 96)	Lunch box selection (page 97) or Vitamin Salad (page 161), 2 slices plain wholemeal bread	Frothy Yogurt Shake (page 98) or small pot low-fat yoghurt	Castilian Fish Soup (page 151)
Tuesday	ACE breakfast choice (page 94)	ACE juice cocktail or ACE fruit snack (page 96)	Lunch box selection (page 97) or Green Bean and Bacon Salad (page 153), jacket potato with 1tsp olive oil	Frothy Yogurt Shake (page 98) or small pot low-fat yoghurt	Almond Pilaff (page 168)
Wednesday	ACE breakfast choice (page 94)	ACE juice cocktail or ACE fruit snack (page 96)	Lunch box selection (page 97) or jacket potato with 1tbsp Hummus (page 144), green salad with 1tbsp dressing	Frothy Yogurt Shake (page 98) or small pot low-fat yoghurt	Pasta Pomodoro (page 174)

Four-week menu plan – Week 1 continued

WEEK 1	Breakfast	Mid-morning snack	Lunch	Tea-time snack	Supper
Thursday	ACE breakfast choice (page 94)	ACE juice cocktail or ACE fruit snack (page 96)	Lunch box selection (page 97) or Fast Fish Risotto (page 180)	Frothy Yogurt Shake (page 98) or small pot low-fat yogurt	Jacket potato with Cucumber and Herb Yogurt (page 160)
Friday	ACE breakfast choice (page 94)	ACE juice cocktail or ACE fruit snack (page 96)	Lunch box selection (page 97) or Stuffed Red Peppers (page 171)	Frothy Yogurt Shake (page 98) or small pot low-fat yoghurt	Greek Spring Salad (page 157)
Saturday	ACE breakfast choice (page 94)	ACE juice cocktail or ACE fruit snack (page 96)	Trimmed Gammon Steak, Pear and Fennel Platter (page 156)	Frothy Yogurt Shake (page 98) or small pot low-fat yogurt	Asparagus with Mushroom Risotto (page 182)
Sunday	ACE breakfast choice (page 94)	ACE juice cocktail or ACE fruit snack (page 96)	Roast Chicken with Apricot Stuffing (page 179), new potatoes, broccoli and carrots. To follow: Strawberry Sorbet (page 192)	Frothy Yogurt Shake (page 98) or small pot low-fat yoghurt	Barley and Vegetable Soup (page 150), with 2 slices plain wholemeal bread

Four-week menu plan

WEEK 2	Breakfast	Mid-morning snack	Lunch	Tea-time snack	Supper
Monday	ACE breakfast choice (page 94)	ACE juice cocktail or ACE fruit snack (page 96)	Lunch box selection (page 97) or Stuffed Courgette Boats (page 175)	Frothy Yogurt Shake (page 98) or small pot low-fat yogurt	Three-Seed Risotto (page 169)
Tuesday	ACE breakfast choice (page 94)	ACE juice cocktail or ACE fruit snack (page 96)	Lunch box selection (page 97) or Frozen Pea Fritters with Passata (page 187)	Frothy Yogurt Shake (page 98) or small pot low-fat yoghurt	Penne with Clams (page 181)
Wednesday	ACE breakfast choice (page 94)	ACE juice cocktail or ACE fruit snack (page 96)	Lunch box selection (page 97) or Vitamin Salad (page 161)	Frothy Yogurt Shake (page 98) or small pot low-fat yogurt	Spinach and Macaroni Pie (page 170)
Thursday	ACE breakfast choice (page 94)	ACE juice cocktail or ACE fruit snack (page 96)	Lunch box selection (page 97) or baked jacket potato with 3oz drained tuna in brine and chopped chives	Frothy Yogurt Shake (page 98) or small pot low-fat yoghurt	Pasta Pomodoro (page 174)

Four-week menu plan – Week 2 continued

WEEK 2	Breakfast	Mid-morning snack	Lunch	Tea-time snack	Supper
Friday	ACE breakfast choice (page 94)	ACE juice cocktail or ACE fruit snack (page 96)	Lunch box selection (page 97) or Three Seed Risotto (page 169)	Frothy Yogurt Shake (page 98) or small pot low-fat yoghurt	Hummus-filled Pitta Pocket (page 144) with Herb Salad (page 154)
Saturday	ACE breakfast choice (page 94)	ACE juice cocktail or ACE fruit snack (page 96)	Black Bean Soup (page 145), Chips in Their Jackets (page 186)	Frothy Yogurt Shake (page 98) or small pot low-fat yoghurt	Prawns with Gazpacho Dressing with brown rice (page 183). To follow: Apricot and Orange Fluff (page 196)
Sunday	ACE breakfast choice (page 94)	ACE juice cocktail or ACE fruit snack (page 96)	Salmon and Sweet Potato Pie with Wilted Greens (page 176). To follow: Spiced Apricots (page 190).	Frothy Yogurt Shake (page 98) or small pot low-fat yoghurt	Tomato and Vegetable Soup (page 146) with 2 slices wholemeal bread

Four-week menu plan

WEEK 3	Breakfast	Mid-morning snack	Lunch	Tea-time snack	Supper
Monday	ACE breakfast choice (page 94)	ACE juice cocktail or ACE fruit snack (page 96)	Lunch box selection (page 97) or Green Bean and Bacon Salad (page 153), jacket potato with 1tsp olive oil (page 142)	Frothy Yogurt Shake (page 98) or small pot low-fat yoghurt	Almond Pilaff (page 168)
Tuesday	ACE breakfast choice (page 94)	ACE juice cocktail or ACE fruit snack (page 96)	Lunch box selection (page 97) or Tuna-stuffed Pitta Pocket (page 141)	Frothy Yogurt Shake (page 98) or small pot low-fat yoghurt	Barley and Vegetable Soup (page 150)
Wednesday	ACE breakfast choice (page 94)	ACE juice cocktail or ACE fruit snack (page 96)	Lunch box selection (page 97) or Vitamin Salad (page 161)	Frothy Yogurt Shake (page 98) or small pot low-fat yoghurt	Pasta Pomodoro (page 174)
Thursday	ACE breakfast choice (page 94)	ACE juice cocktail or ACE fruit snack (page 96)	Lunch box selection (page 97) or Brown Rice and Peanut Salad (page 158)	Frothy Yogurt Shake (page 98) or small pot low-fat yoghurt	Jacket potato with 3oz low-fat cottage cheese and chives

Four-week menu plan – Week 3 continued

WEEK 3	Breakfast	Mid-morning snack	Lunch	Tea-time snack	Supper
Friday	ACE breakfast choice (page 94)	ACE juice cocktail or ACE fruit snack (page 96)	Lunch box selection (page 97) or Barley and Vegetable Soup (page 150)	Frothy Yogurt Shake (page 98) or small pot low-fat yogurt	2 trimmed lamb chops, grilled, with Herbed Mushrooms (page 167)
Saturday	ACE breakfast choice (page 94)	ACE juice cocktail or ACE fruit snack (page 96)	1 egg, scrambled, 2 grilled tomatoes with Healthy Hash Browns (page 185)	Frothy Yogurt Shake (page 98) or small pot low-fat yogurt	Stuffed Red Peppers (page 171)
Sunday	ACE breakfast choice (page 94)	ACE juice cocktail or ACE fruit snack (page 96)	Chicken and Mango Salad (page 159) with Spinach in Yogurt Dressing (page 184). To follow: Strawberry Sorbet (page 192)	Frothy Yogurt Shake (page 98) or small pot low-fat yogurt	Carrot Soup (page 148) followed by Jacket Potato with Cucumber and Tahini filling (page 142)

Four-week menu plan

WEEK 4	Breakfast	Mid-morning snack	Lunch	Tea-time snack	Supper
Monday	ACE breakfast choice (page 94)	ACE juice cocktail or ACE fruit snack (page 96)	Lunch box selection (page 97) or Vitamin Salad (page 161)	Frothy Yogurt Shake (page 98) or small pot low-fat yogurt	Fast Fish Risotto (page 180)
Tuesday	ACE breakfast choice (page 94)	ACE fruit cocktail or ACE fruit snack (page 96)	Lunch box selection (page 97) or Hummus-filled Pitta Pocket (page 144) with Herb Salad (page 154)	Frothy Yogurt Shake (page 98) or small pot low-fat yogurt	Pasta Pomodoro (page 174)
Wednesday	ACE breakfast choice (page 94)	ACE juice cocktail or ACE fruit snack (96)	Lunch box selection (page 97) or Fennel and Pear Platter (page 156)	Frothy Yogurt Shake (page 98) or small pot low-fat yogurt	Stuffed Courgette Boats (page 175)
Thursday	ACE breakfast choice (page 94)	ACE juice cocktail or ACE fruit snack (page 96)	Lunch box selection (page 97) or Greek Spring Salad (page 157)	Frothy Yogurt Shake (page 98) or small pot low-fat yogurt	Penne with Clams (page 181)

Four-week menu plan – Week 4 continued

WEEK 4	Breakfast	Mid-morning snack	Lunch	Tea-time snack	Supper
Friday	ACE breakfast choice (page 94)	ACE juice cocktail or ACE fruit snack (page 96)	Lunch box selection (page 97) or Black Bean Soup (page 145) with Chips in Jackets (page 186)	Frothy Yogurt Shake (page 98) or small pot low-fat yogurt	Asparagus with Mushroom Risotto (page 182)
Saturday	ACE breakfast choice (page 94)	ACE juice cocktail or ACE fruit snack (page 96)	Castilian Fish Soup (page 151)	Frothy Yogurt Shake (page 98) or small pot low-fat yogurt	Spinach and Macaroni Pie (page 170)
Sunday	ACE breakfast choice (page 94)	ACE juice cocktail or ACE fruit snack (page 96)	Grilled turkey steak with Puréed Carrots with Basil (page 188), Red Cabbage and Apple (page 189). To follow: Lemon Meringue (page 195)	Frothy Yogurt Shake (page 98) or small pot low-fat yogurt	Barley and Vegetable Soup (page 150)

7

PREPARING AND COOKING ACE FOODS

Vitality-eating is your best investment for a slim and healthy future

Everyone in the family will benefit from the simple principles of ACE vitality-eating. No matter what age or lifestyle, everybody gains better health, more energy and vitality when they start to eat the ACE way. This chapter outlines the simple steps you need to take to maximize the vitamin values in everyday foods. Once you have completed the twenty-eight-day *Weight-Loss for Life* initial eating plan, you may want to switch to everyday ACE eating. This means following the guidelines of the ACE Plan Pyramid on page 17. ACE vitality-eating means choosing plenty of complex carbohydrates such as wholemeal bread, pasta and potatoes, and lots of ACE vitamin-rich fruits and vegetables. These simple steps guarantee the very best nutrition for those who want healthy, energy-packed meals without necessarily needing to lose more weight. The guidelines in this section apply to all of us – to those just starting the twenty-eight-day *Weight-Loss for Life* eating plan and for those who simply want to maintain their weight-loss and ensure that the pounds don't creep back on. It is also ideal for other members of the family who may not want to follow a weight-loss regime, but who will benefit from the increased vitality and disease-prevention that comes with ACE eating.

ACE Food Shopping

In an ideal world we would get all the vitamins and minerals from our food and not need to take additional supplements. However, it is a sad fact that by the time our food reaches our plates it has already lost many of its valuable ACE vitamins. There are several simple steps we can take to make sure that the vitamins naturally present in foods actually reach our stomachs. The most important point is to avoid over-processed and refined foods as much as possible. For example, wheat flour loses 92 percent of its valuable vitamin E content during the refining process that turns it into white flour, so buy wholemeal flour. Peanuts and almonds lose 80 percent of their vitamin E when they are roasted, so buy them plain.

Some forms of food processing, such as bread-baking and pasta-making are extremely useful, but highly refined foods such as vegetable pizzas, pre-prepared fruit flans and breakfast cereals lose many of their original vitamins. In the case of breakfast cereals, these may be fortified with synthetic vitamins, but these are not as easily absorbed by the body as those naturally present before refining, and give us a false sense of security. Many of the vitamins added in this way also come from animal sources, which may be unacceptable to vegetarians. Most vegetable oils are naturally rich in vitamin E, but some may have had their supplies removed during the refining process. Always choose cold-pressed or unrefined cooking oils which are likely to have more natural vitamin E. As vegetable oils are prone to rancidity it is also worth looking for a use-by date stamp on the bottle before you buy.

When shopping for fruits and vegetables always be guided by your eyes and nose. Reject any produce that looks tired and past its best-by date. Green, leafy vegetables should not be tinged with yellow or brown; pea pods and beans should crisply snap in half and not just bend; while potatoes should be free from shoots and green patches of the poisonous alkaloid solanine. All fruit and vegetables are best bought cold as this is an indication that they have been stored correctly in a cool place. Pre-packed produce kept on the brightly lit shelves of a supermarket will deteriorate faster than produce kept at the back of a dimly lit greengrocer. Don't buy fruit and vegetables that have been on display outside a shop if it is near a road as they will be coated with a thin film of toxic car exhaust fumes. Fruits contain the most beta-carotene when they are ripe. The best way to tell if a beta-carotene rich cantaloupe melon or mango is ripe is to sniff it at the end where it left the stalk. Ripe fruits will smell sweet and fruity when they are ready for eating.

ACE Food Preparation

Always wash fruits and vegetables before eating. This is especially important if the produce has not been organically grown as it is highly likely to have been sprayed with anti-fungal preservatives. As many of these are wax-based, it is worth scrubbing the skins with a nail brush dipped in a weak washing-up liquid solution and thoroughly rinsing before use. Fruit and vegetables begin to oxidize and lose their vitamins the moment they are cut. Aim to leave chopping your fruits and vegetables until the last moment before cooking. The longer they are left open to the light and air, the fewer vitamins they contain. Bags of pre-sliced leeks or ready-grated carrots may be more convenient, but they lose valuable vitamins as they sit under the shop lights.

If you need to prepare vegetables in advance, cut them into larger pieces so that less of their surface area is exposed and store them in a covered container. When preparing dishes such as fresh fruit salad, tightly cover the bowl with clingfilm to reduce the amount of air getting to the fruit and store in a dark place, such as in the fridge. Peeling fruit and vegetables before they are cooked also reduces our levels of ACE vitamins by at least 10 percent. Most of a plant's ACE vitamin supplies are held in its skin near the surface. This is because the antioxidant vitamins protect the plant from burning-up in the sun and without this protection in its skin it would quickly shrivel and die.

ACE Food Cooking

The way we cook our food makes a big difference to vitamin values. It is a well-known fact that over-cooking reduces nutrient levels, but there are also many other factors that affect our food. Of all the nutrients, it is vitamin C that disappears most quickly when food is cooked. This is because vitamin C is water soluble and so it dissolves in the cooking water. A good rule of thumb is to avoid using water whenever possible when cooking fruits and vegetables. A microwave oven is a good investment when it comes to preserving vitamins as the foods are cooked in just a few drops of water. Baking in a conventional oven is also a good form of cooking. For example, a baked jacket potato contains twice as much vitamin C as peeled, boiled potatoes. Steaming vegetables over a pan of boiling water is also a fast and effective way of keeping your valuable vitamins intact. All vegetables can be cooked in this way, even potatoes and other root vegetables.

If you do cook fruits or vegetables in a saucepan of water there are a few golden rules to follow. Always place the food directly into boiling water. This is because the oxidizing enzymes that destroy vitamin C do not work well above temperatures of around 65°C. Putting vegetables into cold water and bringing them slowly to the boil can destroy almost twice as many nutrients. If you opt for boiling your vegetables, use the minimum amount of water necessary. If the vegetables are only a quarter covered by water you will preserve twice as much vitamin C compared to total submersion. Once the vegetables are cooked, don't throw the cooking water down the sink. This coloured cooking liquor is full of energy-giving vitamins that can be kept in the fridge or frozen and used later as a base for a nutritious vegetable stock, soup or gravy.

Beta-carotene is a fat-soluble nutrient, so it is not as easily lost during cooking as vitamin C. Only about 15 percent of beta-carotene is lost during cooking and you can even end up with more beta-carotene from cooked carrots than raw ones. This is because the cooking process breaks down the plant cell walls in fruits and vegetables, increasing the nutrient's availability. For this reason, chopped spinach and puréed carrots have more usual beta-carotene than the raw vegetables. Because beta-carotene is fat soluble, the body absorbs it more easily when it is eaten with a little fat. This does not give us the go-ahead to add spoonfuls of double cream to our fruit salad, but it does mean that cooked carrots can be dabbed with a tiny amount of butter or oil to boost our beta-carotene absorption.

Vitamin E is also a fat-soluble nutrient, so it is best absorbed with a small amount of fat. To maximize our vitamin E values we can eat a small amount of low-fat spread on wholemeal toast, or briefly stir-fry vegetables such as spinach and asparagus in a light spritzing of vegetable oil. Of course, most sources of vitamin E come with their own built-in fat supplies, such as the vegetable oils, avocados, nuts and seeds. Like beta-carotene, vitamin E tends to be fairly stable during the cooking process. The most important point about vitamin E-rich foods is the correct storage to prevent their vitamin E supplies from dwindling before cooking.

Beta-carotene Losses in Cooking
Beta-carotene is stable during most methods of cooking. Canning can decrease the amount of beta-carotene in our food, although in the case of spinach and peas it will actually increase it!

	BETA–CAROTENE – mg per 100g			
Vegetable	**Raw**	**Boiled**	**Frozen and Boiled**	**Canned**
Asparagus	0.32	0.53	–	–
Beans – French	0.33	–	0.18	–
Beans – runner	0.15	0.12	–	–
Beetroot	0.02	0.03	–	–
Broccoli	0.58	0.48	–	–
Cabbage	0.39	0.21	–	–
Carrots – mature	8.12	7.56	–	–
Carrots – young	5.33	4.43	–	–
Courgette	0.61	0.44	–	–
Leeks	7.35	5.75	–	–
Peas	0.3	0.25	0.41	0.06 (processed)
Peppers – green	0.27	0.24	–	–
Peppers – red	3.84	3.78	–	–
Spinach	3.54	3.84	3.84	–
Spring greens	2.63	2.27	–	–
Tomatoes	0.64	–	–	0.22
Fruit	**Raw**	**Stewed**	**Canned in juice**	**Canned in syrup**
Apricots	0.41	–	0.21	0.16
Blackcurrants	0.1	0.08	0.03	0.03
Gooseberries	0.11	0.04	–	0.02
Mango	1.8	–	–	1.5
Plums	0.28	0.06	–	–

	VITAMIN C – mg per 100g			
Vegetable	**Raw**	**Boiled**	**Frozen and Boiled**	**Canned**
Asparagus	12	10	–	–
Beans – French	12	–	7	–
Beans – runner	18	10	–	–
Cabbage – average	49	20	–	–
Carrots	6	2	–	–
Cauliflower	43	27	–	–
Celery	8	4	–	–
Courgette	21	11	–	–
Peas	24	16	12	1
Peas – mange tout	54	28	[stir-fry: 51]	
Peppers – green	120	69	–	–
Peppers – red	140	81	–	–
Potatoes – old	11	6	[roast: 8, baked: 14]	
Potatoes – new	16	15 (without skin: 9)	–	5
Spinach	26	8	6	–
Spring greens	180	77	–	–
Sweet potato	23	17	–	–
Tomatoes	17	–	–	12
Fruit	**Raw**	**Stewed**	**Canned in juice**	**Canned in syrup**
Apple – cooking – peeled	14	11	[unpeeled: 20]	
Apples – eating – average	6	[peeled: 4]		–
Blackberries	15	10	–	–
Blackcurrants	200	115	37	57
Cherries	11	[glacé: trace]		–1
Grapefruit	36	–	33	30
Lychees	45	–	–	8
Peaches	31	–	6	5
Pears	6	–	3	2
Raspberries	32	–	–	7
Strawberries	77	–	–	29

	VITAMIN E – mg per 100g			
Vegetable	**Raw**	**Boiled**	**Canned**	
Asparagus	1.16	1.16	–	
Broccoli	1.3	1.1	–	
Carrots	0.56	0.56	0.64	
Peas	0.21	0.21	0.22	[mushy: 0.3]
Spinach	1.71	1.71	–	
Sweet potato	4.56	4.39	–	
Tomatoes	1.22	–	1.22	
Fruit	**Raw**	**Stewed**	**Canned in juice**	**Canned in syrup**
Apples – eating	0.59	[peeled: 0.27]		–
Blackberries	2.37	2.03	–	–
Blackcurrants	1	0.78	0.54	0.54
Cherries	0.13	[glacé: trace]		0.06
Gooseberries	0.37	0.29	–	0.2
Pears	0.5	[peeled: trace]	Trace	Trace
Raspberries	0.48	–	–	0.15

Boiled vegetables may also contain more beta-carotene than raw as the cooking process releases extra beta-carotene stored in plant cells

Vitamin C Losses in Cooking
Vitamin C is the least stable vitamin during cooking. Canning dramatically reduces vitamin C levels in fruits and vegetables by at least half or more, with the exception of citrus fruits. Peeling potatoes also means throwing away a high proportion of vitamin C.

Vitamin E Losses in Cooking
Vitamin E is very stable during cooking and levels do not significantly change after boiling or canning. However, as vitamin E is affected by heat and light, storage does alter

vitamin E levels. All vitamin E-rich foods, including vegetable oils, should be kept in a cool, dark place and used well within their best-before date.

ACE Food Storage

Careful storage goes a long way in preserving valuable ACE vitamins and makes sure we get the best value for money from our food. Most fruits and vegetables should be stored in a cool, dry place. In today's age of central heating, the bottom drawer of the fridge is the best option if you do not have a cold larder or outside store. Light as well as heat speeds up vitamin losses, so keep your supplies in the dark and not out on display in attractive fruit or vegetable baskets. Once purchased, all fresh produce should be used quickly. It is better to restock fruit and vegetable supplies two or three times a week as the Continentals do. Once opened, fresh fruit juices should also be finished within a few days. This is because oxygen gets into the bottle as soon as the lid is removed and begins to destroy the vitamins. For example, apple juice loses half its vitamin C after four to eight days in the fridge; orange squash loses up to half its vitamin C content within a week of opening the bottle and after three months it may have lost it all. Shaking the bottle or carton of juice, or leaving the container open, also lets more oxygen in and so destroys the vitamins even faster.

Never store chopped vegetables in water as the vitamin C will leak out into the liquid. Once food has been prepared it should be cooked without delay or else tightly covered and stored in the fridge or freezer. The length of storage time also dramatically affects vitamin values. Freshly dug new potatoes contain around 30mg of vitamin C in October, but this drops to around 8mg by the following March. The key to buying fresh produce that really is *fresh* is to buy in season. Most of our everyday crops are seasonal and once harvested, they are put into cold storage for months on end. During this time, vitamin C levels can fall and you can end up with out of season oranges containing no vitamin C at all! If a crop is out of season, you may be better off buying it pre-frozen. Most frozen fruits and vegetables are frozen within an hour of being picked, which means they may well contain more vitamin C than those transported for months of cold storage before ending up under the witheringly bright lights of the supermarket.

As well as the vitamin C and beta-carotene levels lost in fruits and vegetables, Vitamin E is also lost from all cooking oils during storage. This is because vitamin E comes under attack from both light and air. For example, a bottle of safflower oil will have lost more than half its vitamin E content after three months' storage at room temperature. The vitamin E is lost even faster if the bottle is stored on a warm, brightly lit supermarket or kitchen shelf. The best place to store all vegetable oils is in the fridge. Olive oil is slightly more stable as it contains a higher percentage of monounsaturates and so it keeps well in a dark, cool cupboard. All vegetable oils should be used within one month of opening. If you want to preserve your cooking oils for longer and delay rancidity, add the contents of a vitamin E capsule to the bottle and shake well. The extra vitamin E effectively prevents the oil from turning rancid.

Fruit Calendar

January	February	March
Apricots	Apricots	Kumquats
Cranberries	Guavas	Lychees
Guavas	Kumquats	Rhubarb
Lychees	Lychees	
Nectarines	Nectarines	
Peaches	Peaches	
Rhubarb	Rhubarb	
Clementines	Clementines	
Satsumas	Satsumas	

April	May	June
	Gooseberries	Apricots
	Rhubarb	Greengages
	Water melon	Gooseberries
		Nectarines
		Peaches
		Plums
		Raspberries
		Redcurrants
		Rhubarb
		Water melon

July	August	September
Apricots	Blackberries	Blackberries
Blackberries	Damsons	Damsons
Greengages	Greengages	Guavas
Gooseberries	Gooseberries	Nectarines
Nectarines	Guavas	Peches
Peaches	Peaches	Plums
Plums	Peaches	Pomegranates
Raspberries	Plums	Raspberries
Redcurrants	Raspberries	Water melon
Rhubarb	Redcurrants	
Water melon	Water melon	

October	November	December
Bilberries/Blueberries	Guavas	Apricots
Blackberries	Kumquats	Cranberries
Damsons	Lychees	Guavas
Guavas	Nectarines	Lychees
Kumquats	Peaches	Nectarines
Plums	Pomegranates	Peaches
Pomegranates	Raspberries	Raspberries
Raspberries	Sharon fruit	Rhubarb
Satsumas	Clementines	Clementines
Water melon	Satsumas	Satsumas
		Clementines
		Satsumas

	Available all year round	
Avocados	Grapes	Melons
Apples	Grapefruit	Oranges
Bananas	Kiwifruit	Passion fruit
Cherries	Lemons	Pears
Coconuts	Limes	Pineapples
Figs	Mangoes	Strawberries

123

Vegetable Calendar

	Available all year round	
Artichokes Asparagus Aubergines Baby sweetcorn Beans Beansprouts Broccoli Cabbages	Carrots Cauliflower Courgettes Fennel Garlic Leeks Mange tout	Mushrooms Onions Peppers Potatoes Spinach Sweet potatoes Turnips
January	**February**	**March**
Brussels sprouts Kale Parsnips Swedes	Brussels sprouts Kale Parsnips Swedes Sweetcorn	Brussels sprouts Kale Parsnips Swedes Sweetcorn
April	**May**	**June**
Brussels sprouts Kale Marrows Parsnips Swedes Sweetcorn	Kale Marrows Peas Swedes Sweetcorn	Marrows Peas Sweetcorn
July	**August**	**September**
Marrows Peas Sweetcorn	Brussels sprouts Marrows Parsnips Peas Sweetcorn	Brussels sprouts Marrows Parsnips Peas Swedes Sweetcorn
October	**November**	**December**
Brussels sprouts Marrows Parsnips Peas Pumpkins Squash Swedes Sweetcorn	Brussels sprouts Kale Parsnips Pumpkins Squash Swedes	Brussels sprouts Kale Parsnips Swedes
	Available all year round	
Beetroot Celery Chicory Chinese leaves	Chives Cucumbers Lettuce Parsley	Radishes Spring onions Tomatoes Watercress
Celeriac – available from September to April		

ACE Eating-Out

The basic principles of ACE eating for successful weight-loss are less easy to apply when eating away from home. Many of our good intentions and much of our resolve can disappear when we're faced with a restaurant menu. While following the *Weight-Loss for Life* eating plan you are allowed to eat out, provided you stick to the low-fat, ACE menu choices. The golden rule is to avoid anything fried, as this will be overloaded with fat – and our fat cells *love* to feed on fatty foods. The following guidelines will help you enjoy healthy foods without sacrificing your own permanent weight-loss.

British Menus
- Ask for a prawn cocktail without the dressing.
- Minestrone and consommé are low-fat starters.
- Choose boiled or jacket potatoes instead of roast.
- Skip the gravy, choose mint sauce, mustard or herb seasonings instead.
- Don't eat the skin on roast chicken or duck.
- Request plain vegetables without butter.
- Avoid cooked breakfasts, cereal is a lower-fat option.

American Menus
- Hold the mayonnaise and relish on beefburgers.
- Choose a restaurant with a self-service salad bar.
- Use mayonnaise, ketchup and relishes sparingly.
- Choose baked potatoes instead of chips.
- Don't add butter or sour cream.

Chinese Menus
- Fried rice is very high in fat.
- Choose boiled rice which has almost no fat at all.
- Request boiled noodles instead of fried noodles.
- Tofu (beancurd) is a low-fat option.
- Stir-fried vegetables are a good choice.
- Don't be tempted to snack on prawn crackers – they are deep-fried so are high in fat.

- Avoid spring rolls, these also contain a great deal of fat.
- Cashew nuts are high in saturated fat.
- Beansprouts and water chestnuts are a good option.
- Lychees are an excellent, low-fat choice for dessert.

Indian Menus
- Curries can be very high in fat.
- Choose vegetable options and avoid dishes like Chicken Korma which contain cream.
- Indian flat breads are a good choice and better than poppadoms which are deep-fried.
- Basmati rice is an excellent option.
- Avoid deep-fried onion and vegetable bhajis.

Italian Menus
- Minestrone soup, melon and trimmed parma ham are low-fat starters.
- Skinless breast of chicken and grilled fish dishes are a good choice.
- Avoid high-fat Carbonara sauces.
- Choose simple tomato sauce for pasta and only add a small sprinkling of Parmesan cheese.
- Char-grilled vegetables or sea food is a low-fat option.
- Choose sorbet or fresh fruit instead of ice-cream.
- Cappuccino coffee is high in fat, so an espresso is a better choice.

Japanese Menus
- Miso soup with noodles and vegetables is a good choice.
- Soba noodles are made with buckwheat and are low in fat.
- Nori rolls (rice wrapped in seaweed) are deliciously low-calorie. Boiled rice is usually served instead of high-fat fried rice.
- Chicken or beef teriyaki and raw fish sushi are also good, low-fat choices.

Middle Eastern Menus
- Taboullé salad made with cracked wheat and herbs is a good choice.
- Hummus (made without cream) and yogurt dips served with pitta breads are also healthy options.
- Vine leaves stuffed with raisin rice, couscous dishes and savoury lentils are all good choices.
- Avoid deep-fried falalel and samovas.

Top Tips for Eating Out
- Share a starter.
- Order a starter as a main course.
- Ask to be served a smaller portion.
- Request that any nuts, potato chips, bread and butter or bread sticks are removed from the table.
- Always leave some food on your plate.
- Eat half and take a doggy bag home.
- Order plain vegetables with no added butter.
- Most restaurants will serve fresh fruit or a fruit salad for dessert even if it's not on the menu.
- Mix wine with fizzy mineral water to make a spritzer.

The ACE Plan Gourmet

With ideas and recipes like these, no-one will ever guess you are following the ACE *Weight-Loss for Life* eating plan! Exotic fruits, nuts and vegetables are full of vitamins and are useful ingredients when entertaining or cooking to impress. Use good quality, simple ingredients with plenty of colour and texture to create the most impact. Remember that we taste with our eyes as well as our mouths so presentation is all-important.

Exotic ACE Ideas
- The pink-fleshed canteloupe melon not only looks and tastes good, it is also a great source of beta-carotene. Make iced *petits fours* by scooping it into balls with a melon baller. Chill in the freezer for an hour before

serving in a hollowed melon shell. Melon contains plenty of natural sugars which prevents the balls from freezing solid.

- Jars of unsweetened baby food fruit purées are ideal for whipping up an instant fruit coulis. Try varieties such as apricot, strawberry and peach, dilute with a little water and use as a garnish for simple sorbets, frozen yogurt and fruit flans. Alternatively, serve with a fan of sliced fruits such as melon, mango and papaya.

- Turn a simple fruit jelly into a gourmet dessert by adding a dash of sweet white wine to the fruit juices before stirring in the gelatine. Pour over seeded sweet muscat grapes arranged in individual glass dishes dipped in egg-white and sugar.

- Add slices of fresh apple and pineapple to low-calorie coleslaw to get the taste-buds tingling.

- Try using prune purée in place of butter in recipes – to reduce the fat content by 75–90 percent! To make 275g (10oz) of prune purée, blend 225g (8oz) pitted prunes with 6tbsp of water in a food processor until smooth. Prune purée can be used in cake and biscuit baking, and even in savoury recipes.

- Dip fresh strawberries into plain, dark melted chocolate for the (occasional) after-dinner treat. Look out for Green and Black's organic plain chocolate which contains more dark cocoa solids and less added sugar.

- Adding cream to a recipe or pouring it onto a dessert will pile on the calories. Look for lower-fat alternatives, such as low-fat yogurt and fromage frais. Only your waistline will notice the difference.

Fat Facts

Cream		Fromage Frais		Yogurt	
Double	50% fat	Plain	7% fat	Greek	7% fat
Whipping	40%	Fruit	6%	Natural	1.5%
Single	19%	Very low fat	0.5%	Low fat	0.8%

ACE Gourmet Recipes

One of the great advantages with *Weight-Loss for Life* is that you can easily incorporate its principles when it comes to entertaining. The ACE super-slimming foods include many of the more exotic fruits and vegetables that can transform the humblest food into an exotic gourmet dish. Another benefit is that many of these foods are quick and easy to prepare. The following recipes use a variety of the more unusual fresh ingredients to create delicious dishes suitable for entertaining while still following the *ACE Weight-Loss for Life* eating plan.

Gourmet Recipes

Iced almond soup
Cantaloupe soup
Avocado pear with smoked salmon sorbet
Pear and fennel platter
Greek spring salad
Lemon and lambs lettuce salad
Cucumber with herb yogurt
Avocado-raisin dressing
Orange and tamari dressing
Raw apple sauce
Spinach with yogurt dressing
Halibut with watercress sauce
Asparagus and mushroom risotto
Swordfish kebabs
Prawns with gazpacho dressing
Spiced apricots
Walnut apple crisp
Strawberry sorbet
Lemon meringue
Apricot and almond crumble

8

ACE RECIPES

ACE RECIPES

Wake-Up Shake

Serves 2

This wake-up shake will boost your ACE vitamin levels and give you extra energy at the start of the day. It tastes best chilled, so keep your milk or apple juice in the fridge before using. The blackstrap molasses gives the shake a delicious tang and is also a useful source of iron.

1 level tbsp sunflower seeds
1 level tbsp sesame seeds
150ml (¼pt) skimmed milk *or*
150ml (¼pt) apple juice
1 tsp crude blackstrap molasses
1 ripe banana (optional), peeled

PER SERVING:	
Kcals: 350Kc	Beta-carotene: Trace
Fat: 9g (monounsaturated)	Vitamin C: 13.4mg
Fibre: 4.2g	Vitamin E: 7.3mg

Finely grind the seeds in a coffee mill (extra supplies may be ground and stored in the fridge to save preparation time). Blend the ground seeds, milk or apple juice, molasses and banana (if using) together in a food mixer or liquidizer. Serve immediately while still frothy.

Ace Compôte

Serves 4

This compôte is the ideal fast-food breakfast as it is prepared the day before, can be kept in the fridge for at least a week and is ready to serve immediately.

350g (12oz) mixed dried fruit such as:

apple rings	apricots
dates	figs
pears	prunes
raisins	sultanas

½ tsp allspice

½ tsp cinnamon

water

50g (2oz) chopped almonds

PER SERVING:

Kcals: 317Kc	Beta-carotene: 0.2mg
Fat: 7g (monounsaturated)	Vitamin C: 3mg
Fibre: 5.8g	Vitamin E: 3.5mg

Choose unsulphured fruit where possible, preserved without sulphur dioxide. Soak the fruit and spices overnight in 300ml (½pint) water. Serve with plain, live low-fat yogurt and a sprinkling of chopped almonds.

Bircher Muesli

Serves 2

This recipe is based on the original muesli invented by Dr Bircher-Benner for patients at his famous natural health clinic in Switzerland. To save time in the mornings, the oats may be soaked overnight, leaving only the fruit and hazelnuts to be added at breakfast. Dr Bircher-Benner believed that the entire apple should be used – pips and all!

4 tbsp rolled oats
2 tbsp low-fat yogurt
6 tsp cold water
½ tsp grated lemon rind
225g (8oz) freshly grated (unpeeled) apple or 450g (1lb) seasonal soft fruits, such as strawberries
2 tbsp chopped hazelnuts or almonds

PER SERVING:	
Kcals: 163Kc	Beta-carotene: Trace
Fat: 5.5g	Vitamin C: 8.5mg
Fibre: 3.2g	Vitamin E: 2.7mg

Put the oats, yogurt, water and lemon rind into a large bowl and stir until creamy. Leave in the fridge overnight if preferred. Add the fruit and serve sprinkled with the chopped hazelnuts or almonds.

Quick-Cook Wholemeal Bread

Makes 1 large loaf

Wholemeal bread has nearly ten times more vitamin E than white bread. It is also more filling and has far more fibre. My husband learnt to cook this delicious bread at Darina Allen's cookery school at Ballymalloe in Ireland. This recipe is his favourite as it does not need much kneading or proving. Always use organic flour (or conservation grade) when possible as it does not have the pesticide content found in regular wholemeal flour.

450g (1lb) wholemeal flour (Allisons stoneground organic flour is
especially good)
pinch of salt
420ml (scant ¾pt) cold water
1 tsp black treacle
1 sachet dried yeast
1 tsp olive oil to grease loaf tin

PER LOAF:	
Kcals: 1553Kc	Beta-carotene: Nil
Fat: 8.7g (monounsaturated)	Vitamin C: Nil
Fibre: 57g	Vitamin E: 17.8mg

Pre-heat the oven to gas mark 5 (190°C, 375°F).

Place the flour and salt in a large oven-proof bowl and warm in the oven for a few minutes. Stir the black treacle and sachet of dried yeast into 150ml of the water. Warm in the oven to just blood temperature. Stir well and leave the mixture to bubble for 10 minutes. Stir this mixture together with the remaining water into the bowl of flour. Mix well. Brush the insides of a 10-inch loaf tin with olive oil. Place the dough mixture inside the tin and leave in a warm place to rise. After 15–20 minutes, brush the top of the uncooked loaf with the remaining olive oil. Bake for 40–45 minutes. Tip out onto wire rack and allow to cool.

Avocado and Alfalfa Sandwich Filling

Serves 1

A luxurious sandwich recipe which will fill you up with good-ness. Remember to use wholemeal bread for your full quota of Vitamin E.

½ avocado
½ spring onion, finely chopped
dash lemon juice
freshly ground black pepper
large handful alfalfa sprouts (*see below*)
2 thin slices wholemeal bread

PER SERVING:	
Kcals: 241Kc	Beta-carotene: 1.3mg
Fat: 16g (monounsaturated)	Vitamin C: 12.7mg
Fibre: 13g	Vitamin E: 2.1mg

Mash the avocado with the spring onion, lemon juice and black pepper and spread on a slice of bread. Sprinkle with the alfalfa sprouts and top with the second slice of whole-meal bread.

Alfalfa sprouts

These are best eaten shortly after germination as this is when they are at their best. To sprout your alfalfa seeds, place a heaped tablespoon of the seeds in a clean jam jar or pot. Cover the top with a clean, disposable wiping cloth or piece of muslin and secure with an elastic band. Run some cold water into the covered jar, invert it and let the water drain away. Repeat this rinsing several times a day until the seeds have sprouted.

Tahini and Cucumber Sandwich Filling

Serves 1

This is an instant and tasty snack. Tahini spread is made from crushed sesame seeds. It is very high in calcium and is available from good supermarkets and health food shops.

½ tbsp of tahini spread
1 tsp chopped parsley
6 cucumber slices
2 thin slices wholemeal bread

PER SERVING:	
Kcals: 165Kc	Beta-carotene: Trace
Fat: 5g (monounsaturated)	Vitamin C: 31.3mg
Fibre: 1.5g	Vitamin E: 2mg

Spread the tahini spread onto one of the slices of wholemeal bread. Sprinkle the chopped parsley and place the cucumber on top. Serve with cherry tomatoes, radishes and spring onions.

Nut Butter

Nut butter and chopped celery make an unusual and tasty filling for sandwiches and baked potatoes in their jackets. But nut butter is far more versatile than just a spread – try dabbing a little over cooked carrots, or adding ½ teaspoon to a salad dressing for extra flavour. Cashew nuts have the highest fat content, so use sparingly. Hazelnuts are the lowest in fat, while almonds are the richest in vitamin E.

450g (1lb) mixture of almonds, brazil nuts, walnuts, hazelnuts or
peanuts
¼ tsp sea salt
4 tbsp apple juice

PER 25g (1oz) SERVING:

Kcals: 154Kc
Fat: 14g (monounsaturated)
Fibre: 2g

Beta-carotene: Trace
Vitamin C: 0.7mg
Vitamin E: 4mg

Roast the nuts in a medium oven for 10–15 minutes, stirring occasionally. Grind to a fine paste in a coffee mill or food processor with a sharp blade. Dry roast the salt in a pan over a low heat for 1–2 minutes and add to the nut paste. Stir in just enough apple juice to make a thick purée. Store in screw-top jars. If the natural oil in the nuts separates, simply stir it back in. You can also make this recipe using seeds. For seeds such as sesame or sunflower seeds, dry roast in a pan over a low heat until the seeds crush easily when rubbed. Then proceed as before.

Peanut Butter Specials

Peanut butter is a staple sandwich spread. Rich in vitamin E, it works well with many other ingredients to create extra special sandwich fillings.

Try these combinations:
- smooth peanut butter and cucumber
- crunchy peanut butter and celery
- crunchy peanut butter with cottage cheese and pine-apple
- smooth peanut butter and sliced apple
- crunchy peanut butter with alfalfa sprouts and celery

Tuna-Stuffed Pitta Pocket

Serves 1

This tasty combination of tuna and onion makes a light meal or can be packed into a lunch box. Spring onion may be used in place of regular onions.

50g (2oz) tuna, packed in brine
1 tbsp onion, finely chopped
2 tbsp alfalfa sprouts (see page 137)
2 tsp reduced calorie mayonnaise or low-fat fromage frais
1 wholemeal pitta bread
2 lettuce leaves, shredded

PER SERVING:	
Kcals: 253Kc	Beta-carotene: Trace
Fat: 4g (monounsaturated)	Vitamin C: 3.4mg
Fibre: 0.6g	Vitamin E: 0.3mg

Mix together the tuna, onion, alfalfa sprouts and mayonnaise. Slice the pitta bread in half to create two pockets. Line each pocket with shredded lettuce and stuff with the tuna fish mixture.

How to Cook Baked Potatoes

Baked potatoes are the easiest, most economical and versatile of all dishes. If you part-cook them in a microwave oven they are also quick to prepare. It is important to use organically grown potatoes as these are not sprayed with anti-sprouting chemicals or mould inhibitors. You should eat the whole potato, including the skin, as this is where most of the vitamins and fibre are found.

1–2 large potatoes per person, scrubbed clean. Prick the potatoes with a fork and bake in the oven, gas mark 8 (230°C, 450°F) for 1–1½ hours, or until the potatoes have softened inside. Alternatively, place the potatoes in a microwave oven and cook on high for 6–10 minutes, according to size. Place in a hot oven for 10 minutes to crisp the outer skins before serving.

Baked Potato Fillings

Any one of these fillings can be served with a piping-hot potato for lunch or supper as part of your twenty-eight-day weight-loss eating programme.
- *75g (3oz) home-made Hummus (see recipe on page 144)*
- *25g (1oz) Nut Butter and Celery (see page 139)*
- *100g (4oz) Low-fat cottage cheese with chives*
- *1 tsp walnut oil, diced walnuts and celery*
- *2oz grated Edam cheese with fried garlic*
- *½ sliced avocado with sunflower seeds*
- *1 tbsp tahini and dried cucumber*

How to Cook Brown Rice

There are many good reasons for eating brown rice, not least because it tastes great! Much more filling than bland, papery white rice which has had its outer husk and vitamins removed, brown rice also has more fibre, vitamins and minerals. In my experience, the best kind to buy are the organic varieties sold in health food shops. These rices seem to hold their shape and flavour better than the supermarket varieties. Brown rice costs more than white rice because a better quality rice has to be used. However, you are getting your money's worth of important nutrients not found in refined rice.

250g (8oz) assorted brown rices (e.g. Basmati, long grain, short grain)

water

pinch of salt

25g (1oz) sunflower seeds (optional)

PER SERVING (2oz dried):

Kcals: 231Kc	Beta-carotene: Nil
Fat: 1.8g	Vitamin C: Nil
Fibre: 3.6g	Vitamin E: 0.5mg

Wash the rice in a sieve and shake dry. Transfer to a large saucepan, cover with water, approx ¾ inch above the rice. Throw in a pinch of salt and the sunflower seeds (if you are using them). Cover with a lid and bring to the boil. Turn down the heat to a gentle simmer and cook gently for 35–40 minutes, or until soft.

Hummus

Serves 2-4

This is also a delicious filling for sandwiches or baked potatoes, and is very tasty on rye crackers or rice cakes.

50g (2oz) cooked chick peas
juice of 1 lemon
2 cloves garlic, peeled and crushed
1 tbsp cold-pressed olive oil
1 tbsp tahini
50ml (2fl oz) water (optional)

For the garnish:
1 tbsp freshly chopped parsley
1 tbsp pine kernels

PER SERVING:

Kcals: 92Kc	Beta-carotene: Trace
Fat: 5.5g (monounsaturated)	Vitamin C: 37.7mg
Fibre: 2.1g	Vitamin E: 1mg

If using a food processor, place all the ingredients in the bowl and blend until smooth. Alternatively, place all the ingredients in a large mixing bowl and pound with a potato masher, if necessary adding a little water to make the mixture smooth. Serve garnished with parsley and pine nuts.

Spicy Black Bean Soup

Serves 2

A hearty, warming soup that is especially welcome on cold, wet winter evenings. You can use fresh chillies instead of chilli seasoning, but take great care not to rub your eyes before washing the juice from your fingers. Chillies are excellent for clearing the upper respiratory tract and can even unblock the sinuses!

150g (6oz) black-eye beans, cooked
175ml (6fl oz) water or vegetable stock
1 tbsp fresh tomato sauce (see page 174) or 1 tbsp tomato purée
1 tsp chilli seasoning or 1 tsp freshly chopped chillies
1 tsp olive oil (optional)

PER SERVING:

Kcals: 104Kc	Beta-carotene: 0.1mg
Fat: 0.5g	Vitamin C: 6.6mg
Fibre: 3.4g	Vitamin E: Trace

Place the cooked black-eye beans, water or stock, tomato paste and chilli seasoning in a small saucepan. If using fresh chillies, lightly fry in 1 tsp olive oil before adding to the soup. Bring the soup to the boil, turn down the heat and leave to simmer uncovered for 10–15 minutes. Pour about ⅔ of the mixture from the saucepan into a blender and whizz for a few seconds. Return to the remaining ⅓ in the saucepan, heat through and serve.

Tomato and Vegetable Soup

Serves 4

This nourishing soup is quick and easy to make. It has exception-ally high levels of vitamin C and beta-carotene, and is a good nutritional booster for children.

125g (4oz) celery, chopped with its leaves
125g (4oz) carrot, grated
50g (2oz) raw spinach, finely chopped
1ltr (1¾pts) water
125ml (4fl oz) tomato juice
1 tsp honey
½ tsp cayenne pepper
1 tbsp chopped chives

PER SERVING:	
Kcals: 42Kc	Beta-carotene: 6mg
Fat: 0.1g	Vitamin C: 14mg
Fibre: 2.3g	Vitamin E: 0.7mg

Boil the water in a pan and add the chopped vegetables. Cover, turn down the heat and simmer for 20–30 minutes. Add the tomato juice, honey and cayenne pepper. Pour into a blender and liquidize until smooth. Serve with a sprinkling of chopped chives.

Cantaloupe Soup

Serves 4

This chilled soup makes a refreshing starter for a summer dinner party. You can even serve it in the scooped out halves of the melon shell (slice a piece from the bottom to give it a stable base).

2 large, ripe cantaloupe melons
175ml (6fl oz) apple or pear juice
mint leaves to garnish

PER SERVING:	
Kcals: 68Kc	Beta-carotene: 0.9mg
Fat: 0.4g	Vitamin C: 59mg
Fibre: 1g	Vitamin E: Nil

Choose your melons by sniffing, rather than squeezing. A ripe melon will smell ripe at the stalk end, even it feels firm. Slice each melon in half, remove the seeds and discard. Scoop out the flesh and place in a food processor or liquidizer. Add the fruit juice and whizz to a smooth consistency. Chill before serving garnished with mint leaves.

Carrot Soup

Serves 4

This soup is an amazingly good source of beta-carotene, but above all, it tastes delicious! Serve with chunks of freshly baked Quick Cook Wholemeal Bread (see recipe on page 136).

8 large carrots, scrubbed and sliced
1.2ltrs (2pts) water
1 low-salt vegetable stock cube (e.g. Friggs)
1 tbsp chopped coriander or parsley
freshly ground black pepper, to season
scant grating of nutmeg
small carton plain, low-fat yogurt
chopped chives to garnish

PER SERVING:	
Kcals: 72Kc	Beta-carotene: 24mg
Fat: 0.5g	Vitamin C: 33mg
Fibre: 3.6g	Vitamin E: 0.7mg

Cook the carrots in the water with the vegetable stock cube. Add the chopped herbs and seasonings. Purée in a blender or food processor until smooth. Serve in small bowls with a swirl of plain yogurt and a sprinkling of chopped chives to garnish.

Beetroot Soup

Serves 4

675g (1lb) steamed beetroot
1 tsp fennel seeds
2 cloves of garlic, crushed
2 tbsp olive oil
½ltr (1pt) water
2 tbsp low-fat fromage frais
1 tbsp freshly chopped mint

PER SERVING:	
Kcals: 90Kc	Beta-carotene: 2.5mg
Fat: 0.9g	Vitamin C: 41.2mg
Fibre: 0.7g	Vitami E: 0.5mg

Roughly chop the beetroot and lightly fry in the olive oil. Add the crushed garlic and sprinkle with fennel seeds. Pour in the water, season with salt and pepper, and cover the pan with a lid. Turn down the heat and leave the soup to simmer for 10–15 minutes. Remove it from the heat and liquidize to a smooth purée. Serve in individual bowls with a spoonful of fromage frais garnished with chopped mint.

Barley and Vegetable Soup

Serves 4

A hearty, nourishing soup that satisfies the hungriest of stomachs. This recipe works particularly well with root vegetables, such as carrot, parsnip and swede.

3 tbsp cold-pressed olive oil
2 onions, peeled and chopped
450g (1lb) any colourful vegetable, chopped, diced or shredded
75g (3oz) pot barley
½ tsp freshly grated root ginger
1.2ltrs (2pts) vegetable stock
freshly ground pepper

PER SERVING:	
Kcals: 190Kc	Beta-carotene: 8.2mg
Fat: 1.5g	Vitamin C: 16.6mg
Fibre: 9g	Vitamin E: 1.1mg

In a large saucepan, heat the oil and lightly sauté the onions and the other vegetable of your choice. Stir in the pot barley, root ginger and stock, and season with the freshly ground black pepper. Cover and simmer over a low heat for 2 hours or until the barley is soft.

Castilian Fish Soup

Serves 4-6

This hearty Spanish soup is both nutritious and filling, and makes a delicious one-course meal. It is also a good way of using up leftover rice. Alternatively, use Whole Earth's pre-cooked tinned brown rice which has a good flavour and is a great time-saver.

1kg (2lb) firm-fleshed fish, e.g. cod, hoki or hake
1ltr (1¾pts) water
2 tbsp olive oil
3 cloves garlic, crushed
1 medium onion, chopped
8 large tomatoes, chopped
1 red pepper, de-seeded and chopped
salt and pepper
½kg (1lb) new potatoes, scrubbed
300g (11oz) cooked brown rice
50g (2oz) parsley, finely chopped

PER SERVING:	
Kcals: 441Kc	Beta-carotene: 1.4mg
Fat: 4.8g	Vitamin C: 82mg
Fibre: 6.7g	Vitamin E: 2.5mg

Briefly fry the fish in 1tbsp of the olive oil. Flake into large chunks and remove any bones. Place the bones in a saucepan with the water, the remaining olive oil, garlic, onion, tomatoes and seasoning. Bring to the boil, cover and simmer for 30–40 minutes. Strain the liquid through a sieve and add the new potatoes. Simmer gently for 20 minutes or until the potatoes have softened. Add the cooked brown rice and adjust the seasoning. Just before serving, stir in the pieces of fish and sprinkle with freshly chopped parsley.

Iced Almond Soup

Serves 4

This deliciously refreshing summer soup tastes best when using freshly ground almonds. Commercially ground almonds may be used if you're in a hurry, but these are prone to rancidity and vitamin E loss. Almonds can easily be ground in their skins using a coffee grinder or with the sharp blade of a food mixer. This recipe is an especially good source of vitamin E.

2 slices wholemeal bread without crusts
275ml (1pt) cold water
2 cloves garlic, peeled and freshly crushed
100g (4oz) finely ground almonds
2 tbsp olive oil
2 tbsp fresh lemon juice
salt to season
4 sprigs of fresh mint

PER SERVING:

Kcals: 179Kc	Beta-carotene: 1.5mg
Fat: 13g (monounsaturated)	Vitamin C: 13.6mg
Fibre: 2.4g	Vitamin E: 6.3mg

Crumble the bread into a food processor, pour on half the water, add the garlic and almonds, and whizz until smooth. Pour the olive oil and lemon juice into the remaining water and dribble this mixture into the food processor while it is still going. The soup should take on the consistency of thin yogurt. Season with salt to taste before chilling in the fridge for at least an hour. Serve in small bowls decorated with chopped mint.

Green Bean and Bacon Salad

Serves 4

This colourful salad makes a tasty light lunch or a good accompaniment to a baked jacket potato.

450g (1lb) green beans, trimmed and sliced into 1½in lengths
4 rashers lean bacon
1 red pepper, de-seeded and roughly chopped
1 small onion, finely chopped

For the dressing:
150ml (5fl oz) natural, low-fat yogurt
1 tbsp olive oil
1 tbsp lemon juice
1 tsp Dijon mustard
2 tbsp chopped chives
1 clove garlic, crushed
freshly ground black pepper

PER SERVING:

Kcals: 154Kc	Beta-carotene: 0.3mg
Fat: 3g	Vitamin C: 28mg
Fibre: 3g	Vitamin E: 0.5mg

Steam or microwave the beans in a small amount of water until tender, but still crisp. Trim the fatty rind off the bacon and grill. Cut into bite-sized pieces. Mix the beans, bacon and chopped raw onion and red pepper together. Stir all the dressing ingredients together and whisk. Pour the dressing over the leaves and stir well.

Herb Salad

Serves 4

This tasty all-leaf salad makes a great accompaniment to pasta. Don't be tempted to make a more complicated dressing but let the herb flavours speak for themselves.

300g (11oz) mixed salad leaves such as:

spinach	radiccio
frisee	chicory
rocket (arugula)	

50g (2oz) watercress

50g (2oz) mixed fresh herb leaves such as:

chervil	basil
parsley	coriander

2 tbsp olive oil or walnut oil

1 tsp lemon juice

PER SERVING:	
Kcals: 26Kc	Beta-carotene: 2.4mg
Fat: 0.7g	Vitamin C: 43.3mg
Fibre: 2g	Vitamin E: 1.3mg

Toss all the ingredients together and serve.

Lemon and Lambs Lettuce Salad

Serves 4 as a starter or side salad

This light salad makes a refreshing change in the summer months and is a good accompaniment to cold chicken or fish dishes.

100g (4oz) lambs lettuce, trimmed
100g (4oz) watercress, roughly chopped
1 lemon (unwaxed)
2 tbsp extra virgin olive oil
black pepper
6 radishes, trimmed and sliced

PER SERVING:	
Kcals: 14Kc	Beta-carotene: 0.4mg
Fat: 0.6g	Vitamin C: 30mg
Fibre: 0.7g	Vitamin E: 0.4mg

Mix the lambs lettuce and chopped watercress together in a serving bowl. Wash the lemon and finely slice into small pieces. Briefly blanch in boiling water until the peel softens. Add the blanched lemon pieces to the bowl, together with a sprinkling of freshly ground black pepper and olive oil. Mix well. Arrange the radish slices on top of the salad as an attractive garnish.

Pear and Fennel Platter

Serves 4 as a starter or side dish

This simple salad uses an unusual combination of readily available, fresh ingredients. Leave the peel on the pears to maximize their vitamin value.

2 bulbs of fennel, trimmed
2 ripe pears
100g (4oz) Edam, Emmenthal or Gouda cheese
50g (2oz) finely chopped fresh parsley
1 tbsp extra virgin olive oil

PER SERVING:	
Kcals: 162Kc	Beta-carotene: Trace
Fat: 7g	Vitamin C: 56mg
Fibre: 2.3g	Vitamin E: 0.1mg

Cut the fennel bulbs into thick slices and blanch by plunging into boiling water for 15–20 seconds. Wash the pears and chop them into thin slices, removing the core and pips. Use a cheese-slicer or sharp knife to carve the cheese into wafer-thin slices. Arrange the blanched fennel, pear pieces and cheese on a large platter. Sprinkle with chopped parsley and drizzle with drops of best quality olive oil.

Greek Spring Salad

Serves 4

Baby spinach is a good choice for this light salad. Feta cheese can be substituted for the cottage cheese, but it has a much higher fat content.

450g (16oz) raw spinach
175g (6oz) cottage cheese
50g (2oz) currants
50g (2oz) black olives, pitted
50g (2oz) radishes, thinly sliced
4 spring onions, sliced lengthways

For the dressing:
2 tbsp sunflower oil
1 tbsp lemon juice
1 tbsp sesame seeds
1 clove garlic, crushed and chopped
1 tsp fresh oregano, chopped
salt and black pepper

PER SERVING:	
Kcals: 175Kc	Beta-carotene: 7mg
Fat: 12g (monounsaturated)	Vitamin C: 63mg
Fibre: 4.5g	Vitamin E: 4.1mg

Rinse the spinach and dry it. Tear the larger leaves into bite-sized pieces, discarding any stringy stems. Place in a large salad bowl, add the cheese, currants, black olives and radishes. Mix the dressing ingredients together and pour over the salad. Toss well and garnish with the spring onions.

Brown Rice and Peanut Salad

Serves 4-6

This nutty flavoured salad is wonderful for a light summer supper and also works well as a side-dish with smoked fish or cold cuts of meat.

500g (10oz) brown rice, cooked
75g (3oz) peanuts, unsalted
75g (3oz) currants
50g (2oz) sunflower seeds
4 spring onions, finely sliced
2 tbsp parsley, chopped (reserve a few sprigs for garnishing)
1 dark lettuce, washed and trimmed

For the dressing:
2 tbsp sunflower oil
2 tbsp cider or white wine vinegar
2 tsp Dijon mustard
2 cloves garlic, crushed and chopped
½ tsp dried thyme
salt and black pepper

PER SERVING:	
Kcals: 329Kc	Beta-carotene: 2mg
Fat: 19g (monounsaturated)	Vitamin C: 65mg
Fibre: 4.5g	Vitamin E: 8.1mg

In a large bowl, toss the cooked brown rice with the peanuts, currants, sunflower seeds, spring onions and parsley. Mix the dressing ingredients together and pour over the rice salad. Stir well. Serve the salad in a lettuce-lined bowl, sprinkled with chopped parsley.

Chicken and Mango Salad

Serves 6

This is a delicious dish for a summer lunch or light supper. In the unlikely event of any being left over, use to stuff pitta bread or serve warm on a bed of brown rice.

1 medium-size free-range chicken
1 medium onion, peeled and roughly chopped
1 ripe mango
small bunch seedless grapes
4 spring onions

For the dressing:
85ml (3fl oz) sunflower or safflower oil
1 tbsp white wine or cider vinegar
1 tsp honey
1 tbsp plain, low-fat, live yogurt
salt and black pepper

PER SERVING:	
Kcals: 415Kc	Beta-carotene: 2.5mg
Fat: 22.4g	Vitamin C: 17.8mg
Fibre: 2.1g	Vitamin E: 0.2mg

Not only are free-range chickens more kindly reared, they also taste better. First, rinse the bird inside and out before placing in a large saucepan half filled with simmering water. Add the chopped onion for added flavour, cover the pan and leave to cook gently for approximately 1½ hours. Test to see if the chicken is cooked by piercing the thigh area with a sharp knife or skewer. The juice should run clear when it is ready. Remove the chicken from the pan and cool rapidly. Do not leave the chicken in a warm place for more time than necessary as this encourages bacteria to breed. When cold, remove the meat from the carcass keeping the pieces as large as possible. Skin the meat (most of the fat is in the skin) and cut into bite-sized chunks.

Peel the mango and cut into cubes roughly the same size as the chicken pieces. Wash the grapes and remove the stalks. Wash and trim the spring onions before finely slicing them. Add to the chicken pieces and mix together in a large bowl. Make the dressing by whisking all the ingredients together in a jug or bowl. Alternatively, put all the ingredients into a screw-top jar and shake well to mix. Pour the dressing over the chicken salad and toss with a spoon. Serve on wholemeal pasta cooked in the chicken stock or new potatoes still in their skins.

Cucumber with Herb Yogurt

Serves 4

A simple side dish to accompany lean cold meats or seafood. Similar to the Indian raita, this dish can be served as a snack with chapatis, wholemeal bread or rye crackers.

2 cucumbers
50g (2oz) each of fresh parsley and mint, finely chopped
175ml (6fl oz) plain, low-fat, live yogurt
1 lime
salt and black pepper

PER SERVING:	
Kcals: 57Kc	Beta-carotene: 2.5mg
Fat: 1g	Vitamin C: 42.8mg
Fibre: 0.1g	Vitamin E: Nil

Wash the cucumbers and trim the ends. Chop into bite-sized chunks. Place in a large bowl together with the herbs and yogurt. Stir well. Squeeze the juice from the lime and add. Season with salt and pepper before serving.

Vitamin Salad

This salad can be adapted to include any of your favourite vegetables. All the vegetables should be raw.

50g (2oz) Brussels sprouts, grated
50g (2oz) parsnip, peeled and grated
50g (2oz) carrot, scrubbed and grated
50g (2oz) swede, peeled and grated
50g (2oz) raw beetroot, grated
50g (2oz) radishes, trimmed and thinly sliced
50g (2oz) olives, finely diced
50g (2oz) cabbage, shredded
50g (2oz) celery, chopped
1 small onion, peeled and finely chopped
50g (2oz) watercress or mustard and cress
salad dressing of your choice

PER SERVING:	
Kcals: 75Kc	Beta-carotene: 2.5mg
Fat: 1.7g	Vitamin C: 38.2mg
Fibre: 2.8g	Vitamin E: 0.02mg

Mix all the ingredients together in a large bowl and stir in your favourite dressing.

Yogurt and Chive Dressing

Serves 2-4

This tangy dressing is good for leafy salads, baked potatoes or for turning leftover pasta or rice into a salad dish.

150ml (¼pt) natural, low-fat, live yogurt
1 tbsp cold-pressed olive oil
1 tbsp lemon juice
1 tsp Dijon mustard
2 tbsp chopped chives
1 clove garlic, peeled and crushed
freshly ground black pepper

PER SERVING:	
Kcals: 35Kc	Beta-carotene: Trace
Fat: 1g	Vitamin C: 3.4mg
Fibre: Trace	Vitamin E: 0.1mg

In a large bowl, mix all the ingredients together, adding the black pepper, and stir vigorously. Alternatively, place the ingredients in a large screw-top jar, replace the lid and shake well.

Orange and Tamari Dressing

Serves 2-4

This is very good with green-leafed vegetables such as raw spinach or salad leaves. It is also a useful dressing for those who dislike using vinegar.

150ml (¼pt) freshly squeezed orange juice
1 tsp grated orange peel
2 tbsp tamari sauce
1 tsp finely chopped fresh root ginger
3 tbsp cold-pressed olive oil
1 clove garlic, peeled and crushed

PER SERVING:	
Kcals: 40Kc	Beta-carotene: Trace
Fat: 0.9g	Vitamin C: 27mg
Fibre: 0.4g	Vitamin E: 0.8mg

In a large bowl, mix all the ingredients together and stir well before using. Alternatively, place the ingredients in a large, screw-top jar, replace the lid and shake well.

Raw Apple Sauce

Serves 2-4

This is a recipe which has many different uses. Serve the sauce cold as an accompaniment to lean, grilled pork chops or cold cuts of chicken and turkey. This sauce is also great served warm with plain low-fat frozen yogurt and an extra sprinkling of cinnamon.

4 eating apples, cored and chopped (preferably unpeeled
juice of ½ lemon
a little grated nutmeg
a pinch of cinnamon
50-100ml (2–4fl oz) apple juice

PER SERVING:	
Kcals: 123Kc	Beta-carotene: Trace
Fat: 0.6g	Vitamin C: 13mg
Fibre: 4g	Vitamin E: 1.2mg

Blend the apples with the lemon juice and spices in a food processor. Add sufficient apple juice to achieve the desired consistency. The sauce may be warmed through gently in a small saucepan if preferred, but do not let it boil.

Avocado-Raisin Dressing

Serves 2-4

This textured dressing is perfect poured over baked potatoes, crisp green salads or sliced tomatoes.

1 large ripe avocado
1 tbsp lemon juice
50g (2oz) seedless raisins
50g (2oz) low-fat fromage frais
salt and black pepper to season

PER SERVING:	
Kcals: 156Kc	Beta-carotene: Trace
Fat: 11g (monounsaturated)	Vitamin C: 9.5mg
Fibre: 9.2g	Vitamin E: 1.4mg

Peel the avocado, remove the stone (keep to one side) and mash with a potato masher or fork. Stir in the remaining ingredients and mix well. Place in a serving dish with the avocado stone in the centre to help prevent discolouring. Remove the stone just before serving.

Avocado Pear with Smoked Salmon Sorbet

Serves 4

This is an impressive starter for any dinner. The sorbet needs to be prepared the day before serving and can be made with smoked salmon scraps which are much cheaper than slices.

For the sorbet:
100g (4oz) smoked salmon pieces
4 tbsp low-fat fromage frais
1 tsp horseradish sauce
2 tbsp lemon juice
salt and black pepper

To serve:
2 large ripe avocado pears
1 tbsp lemon juice
4 sprigs of basil

PER SERVING:	
Kcals: 182Kc	Beta-carotene: Trace
Fat: 17g (monounsaturated)	Vitamin C: 15mg
Fibre: 12.8g	Vitamin E: 2.1mg

Make the sorbet the day before by blending all the ingredients together in a food processor. Pour into a bowl or freezer container and freeze for 8 hours occasionally stirring the mixture. Remove from the freezer 15–20 minutes before serving. Cut the avocados in half and remove the stone and peel. Slice the avocado halves lengthways and transfer to a plate. Fan out the avocado slices and brush with lemon juice to avoid discolouration. Place two scoops of salmon sorbet on each place and garnish with a sprig of basil. Serve immediately.

Herbed Mushrooms

Serves 4–6

These mushrooms are delicious served alone as a starter or as a salad ingredient. They can also be drained and served warm as a vegetable side dish.

450g (1lb) mushrooms
250ml (8fl oz) red wine vinegar
100g (4oz) onions, finely chopped
1tsp mixed spice, pickling spice or allspice
4 cloves
100g (4oz) red pepper, de-seeded and sliced
120ml (4fl oz) sunflower oil
salt and pepper

PER SERVING:	
Kcals: 120Kc	Beta-carotene: Trace
Fat: 5.0g (monounsaturated)	Vitamin C: 13.25mg
Fibre: 1.83g	Vitamin E: 0.4mg

Lightly brush the mushrooms with a damp cloth to re-move any earth. Blanch by plunging briefly into boiling water for 20 seconds. Drain and allow to cool. Meanwhile, bring the vinegar to boil in a non-aluminium pan. Add the chopped onions and seasonings. Cook for 2–3 minutes before adding the chopped red peppers, sunflower oil and salt and pepper. Cool the mixture, add the mushrooms and leave to marinade for 2–3 hours. Drain the oil and juices before serving. The mushrooms can be stored in a screw-top jar in the refrigerator for at least a fortnight.

ACE Tip: Drain the seasoned oil from the mushrooms before serving to reduce their fat content.

Almond Pilaff

Serves 4

This is a delicious, nutty dish that is both light and filling. Eat on its own or serve as a side-dish with meat or fish.

150g (5oz) millet
1 tbsp olive oil
1 medium onion, finely chopped
1 carrot, scrubbed and chopped
2 cloves garlic, crushed and chopped
small piece root ginger, grated
100g (4oz) whole almonds
350ml (12fl oz) water
150g (6oz) brown rice, cooked
salt and black pepper

PER SERVING:	
Kcals: 366Kc	Beta-carotene: 3.04mg
Fat: 15g (monounsaturated)	Vitamin C: 6.3mg
Fibre: 10g	Vitamin E: 7.3mg

Place the millet in a large saucepan and stir it over a moderate heat until it begins to toast and the grains pop open. Transfer the millet to a plate. Heat the oil in the saucepan and add the onion, carrot, garlic and grated ginger root. Cook until the onion is translucent and the carrots have softened. Meanwhile, rinse the almonds and dry-roast in a pan over a high heat. Add the toasted millet to the vegetable mixture, pour in the water and bring to the boil. Cover and simmer over a low heat for 15–20 minutes or until all the water has been absorbed and the millet is cooked. Stir in the pre-cooked brown rice and warm through. Sprinkle with toasted almonds and serve hot.

Three-Seed Risotto

Serves 4-6

I make plenty of this risotto as it keeps well in the fridge for 4-5 days. I then use it as a base for vegetable risottos or add it to soups and casseroles. It is also a favourite with my children and can be mixed with vegetable purées for a toddler's tea.

150g (6oz) long grain organic brown rice
75g (3oz) millet
50g (2oz) sunflower seeds (without shells)
1 tbsp olive oil
1 medium onion, finely diced
2 cloves garlic, crushed and chopped
1 low-salt vegetable stock cube (eg Friggs)
900ml (1½pint) water
1 tbsp low-salt yeast extract
1 tbsp parsley, chopped

PER SERVING:	
Kcals: 264Kc	Beta-carotene: Trace
Fat: 6g (monounsaturated)	Vitamin C: 20mg
Fibre: 5g	Vitamin E: 5.4mg

Rinse the grains and seeds in a sieve under cold running water and shake dry. Heat the oil in a frying pan and lightly sauté the onion and garlic until translucent. Add the mixed grains and stir for 2–3 minutes. Heat the water and dissolve the stock cube and yeast extract in it. Transfer to a large saucepan. Add the mixed grains and bring to the boil. Reduce the heat, cover and simmer for 30–35 minutes or until the rice has cooked through. Sprinkle with chopped parsley and serve.

ACE Tip: This is a great base for many other grain dishes. Try adding vegetables or chopped tomatoes.

Spinach and Macaroni Pie

Serves 4

This tasty pasta pie freezes well, so make an extra one for the freezer. If you can't find fresh spinach, use a block of frozen spinach which has just as many vitamins and also cuts down the preparation time. This recipe is a great source of all three ACE vitamins.

300g (11oz) dried wholewheat macaroni
450g (1lb) fresh spinach or 225g (8oz) block of frozen spinach, thawed
50ml (2fl oz) skimmed milk
1 medium onion, chopped
3 cloves garlic, crushed and chopped
small piece root ginger, grated
100g (4oz) wholewheat breadcrumbs
50g (2oz) parmesan cheese, grated
25g (1oz) sesame seeds

PER SERVING:	
Kcals: 472Kc	Beta-carotene: 4.5mg
Fat: 9g (monounsaturated)	Vitamin C: 36.4mg
Fibre: 10g	Vitamin E: 5.2mg

Pre-heat the oven to gas mark 5 (190°C, 375°F).

Cook the macaroni according to the instructions on the packet. Rinse in cold water to stop the cooking process and drain. If using fresh spinach, wash it and chop it into small pieces. Cook in boiling water for 2–3 minutes. Place the spinach in a large mixing bowl. Add the milk, onion, garlic, grated ginger root to season. Stir in the cooked macaroni and transfer to a baking dish. Mix together the breadcrumbs, parmesan cheese and sesame seeds. Sprinkle liberally over the macaroni mixture. Bake in a pre-heated oven for 20–25 minutes or until the breadcrumb topping is crisp and golden.

Stuffed Red Peppers

Serves 4

A no-fuss supper dish that looks impressive but takes no time to put together. Serve with spring greens or spinach.

4 large red peppers
1 medium onion, finely chopped
50ml (2fl oz) olive oil
100g (4oz) grated carrot
200g (7oz) long grain brown rice
600ml (1pt) vegetable or chicken stock
275g (10oz) packet of frozen peas
75g (3oz) seedless raisins
½ tsp dried thyme
salt and pepper to season
1 tbsp parsley, chopped
50g (2oz) slivered almonds, toasted

PER SERVING:	
Kcals: 584Kc	Beta-carotene: 4.8mg
Fat: 14g (monounsaturated)	Vitamin C: 73.4mg
Fibre: 11g	Vitamin E: 4mg

Pre-heat the oven to gas mark 5 (190°C, 375°F).

In a large pan lightly fry the onion in the olive oil, add the carrot and rice, stir well. Pour in the stock, add the peas, raisins, thyme, and salt and pepper. Prepare the peppers by removing their stalks (push the stalks down into the pepper, twist and remove). Rinse the seeds out from inside each one. Slice a piece from the bottom of each pepper so they stand securely. Place on a non-stick baking sheet and bake in the pre-heated oven for 15–20 minutes. Remove from the oven and stuff with the rice mixture. Sprinkle with the chopped parsley and toasted almonds. Serve hot.

Halibut with Watercress Sauce

Serves 4

Halibut is ideal for baking because it can be cut like a steak, has a firm texture and doesn't fall apart as you transfer it to a plate. A whole halibut can weigh up to 300 pounds, which means that the steaks are large enough to satisfy the heartiest appetites.

1 small onion, finely chopped
150ml (¼pt) dry white wine
1kg (approx 2lb) halibut steaks
1 tbsp olive oil
100g (4oz) watercress, chopped
1 tsp smooth mustard
salt and pepper

PER SERVING:

Kcals: 324Kc	Beta-carotene: 0.7mg
Fat: 6g	Vitamin C: 18mg
Fibre: 1.2g	Vitamin E: 0.3mg

Pre-heat the oven to Gas mark 8 (230°C, 450°F).

Place the onions and white wine in a casserole dish or stainless steel baking pan (with a lid). Lay the halibut steaks on top and drizzle with olive oil. Cover and bake in the pre-heated oven for 15–20 minutes until almost cooked through. Move the fish to a hot serving dish and cover with a lid or a piece of foil to keep warm. Transfer the cooking juices to a small saucepan, add the chopped watercress and boil on a high heat for about a minute. Use a hand-held blender (or transfer to a food processor) to purée the sauce until smooth. Add the mustard, salt and pepper to taste and pour over the halibut just before serving.

Swordfish Kebabs

Serves 4

These are all-year favourites, but taste especially good barbecued over a charcoal grill in the summer. Swordfish is increasingly available from fish counters, but can be substituted with king prawns or sea scallops.

2 tbsp freshly squeezed lemon juice
4 tbsp olive oil
1 tsp mixed dried herbs
1 tsp whole grain mustard
salt and black pepper
750g (1½lb) swordfish, cubed (about 24 pieces)
100g (4oz) button mushrooms
4 medium onions, quartered
2 red peppers, cubed
8 ripe cherry tomatoes

PER SERVING:	
Kcals: 437Kc	Beta-carotene: 0.6mg
Fat: 11g (monounsaturated)	Vitamin C: 54mg
Fibre: 6.202g	Vitamin E: 1.6mg

Place the lemon juice, oil and seasonings in a large bowl and mix well. Add the fish and chopped vegetables and toss well. Leave to marinade for at least one hour. Pre-heat the grill. Assemble the kebabs, allowing 2 skewers per person. Place under the grill, brush with the remaining marinade and cook for 6–8 minutes, turning occasionally to prevent the vegetables burning. Serve with brown rice or baked jacket potatoes.

Pasta Pomodoro

Serves 6-8

This rich tomato sauce can be used for pasta, rice or even leftover fish. I always make twice the quantity as it keeps for up to a week in the fridge or in the freezer for three months. Passata (sieved tomatoes) is a good substitute for whole tomatoes and works well in this recipe. Carton or jars of passata can be found in most supermarkets.

For the sauce:
120ml (4fl oz) olive oil
300g (10oz) onion, finely chopped
100g (4oz) carrot, chopped
4 cloves garlic, crushed
1kg (2¼lb) tomatoes, chopped *or* 1ltr (1¾ pint) passata
1 tbsp basil, chopped
1 tbsp oregano, chopped

Pasta:
Allow 100g (4oz) dried wholemeal pasta per person

PER SERVING:	
Kcals: 412Kc	Beta-carotene: 3.4mg
Fat: 3g	Vitamin C: 32mg
Fibre: 6g	Vitamin E: 1.1mg

Heat the oil in a large saucepan or deep-sided frying pan. Add the onions, carrot and garlic. Stir frequently until the vegetables have softened. Add the chopped tomatoes or passata, cover the pan and simmer over a low heat for 20 minutes. Stir in the chopped herbs, partially cover and simmer for a further 10 minutes.

Cook the pasta until al dente (slightly firm), drain and serve immediately with a helping of pomodoro sauce. Sprinkle with freshly grated parmesan cheese (optional).

Stuffed Courgette Boats

Serves 4

This is a quick and tasty way to use up the summer glut of cour-gettes. Serve with baby new potatoes or brown rice cooked in vegetable stock for added flavour.

2 large courgettes
1 small onion, finely chopped
50g (2oz) celery, finely chopped
2 cloves garlic, crushed and chopped
75ml (2fl oz) tomato juice
1 small slice wholemeal bread
1 tbsp wholemeal breadcrumbs
1 tsp dried mixed herbs

PER SERVING:	
Kcals: 54Kc	Beta-carotene: 0.2mg
Fat: 0.2g	Vitamin C: 11mg
Fibre: 1.7g	Vitamin E: 0.3mg

Pre-heat the oven to gas mark 4 (180°C, 350°F).

Steam or microwave the courgettes until just cooked. Cut them lengthwise and scoop out the centres. Mix together the centre pulp with the onion, celery and garlic. Soak the slice of wholemeal bread in the tomato juice before mashing it and adding to the mixture. Add half the breadcrumbs and herbs, and season with salt and pepper. Mix well before stuffing the courgette boats. Sprinkle with the remaining breadcrumbs and bake for 30–40 minutes.

Salmon and Sweet Potato Pie with Wilted Greens

Serves 4

This is one of my family's favourites and it is so easy to serve as you bake the sweet potato together with the fish. This dish is a real nutritional winner too, as it is low in calories and high in all three ACE vitamins.

200g (8oz) fresh salmon steaks
1 tbsp fresh lemon juice
1 tbsp fresh dill, chopped
salt and black pepper
100g (4oz) wholewheat pasta shells, cooked and drained
1 tbsp olive oil
(4fl oz) skimmed milk
200g (8oz) cooked, mashed sweet potatoes
50g (2oz) toasted sunflower seeds
1 tsp olive oil for greasing baking dish

For the greens:
350g (12oz) fresh spinach or spinach greens
1 tsp freshly grated ginger root
1 tsp soya or tamari sauce

PER SERVING:	
Kcals: 285Kc	Beta-carotene: 8.5mg
Fat: 12g (monounsaturated)	Vitamin C: 36.6mg
Fibre: 5g	Vitamin E: 5.2mg

Pre-heat the oven to gas mark 5 (190°C, 375°F).

Place the salmon in a baking dish, sprinkle with lemon juice, dill and salt and pepper to season. Cover and bake for 15 minutes, or until cooked. Flake the fish and set aside. Mix together the skimmed milk and olive oil, stir in the sweet potatoes and mix well. Add the pre-cooked pasta, flaked salmon pieces and toasted sunflower seeds. Oil the baking dish to prevent the mixture from sticking. Pour the mixture into the dish, cover and bake in the oven for 20 minutes.

Prepare the wilted greens by washing and trimming any tough stalks. Place in a steamer over a pan of boiling water, sprinkle with ginger root and lightly steam for 5–10 minutes. Remove from the pan, sprinkle with soya sauce and serve with the pie.

Really Easy Roast Chicken

It's not much more fiddly to include the Apricot Stuffing but I'll leave the choice to you.

1 fresh free-range chicken
1 tbsp cold-pressed olive oil
2 tbsp chopped, fresh mixed herbs or 1 tbsp dried mixed herbs
freshly ground black pepper
1 recipe quantity Apricot Stuffing (see page 179)

PER SERVING:	
Kcals: 564Kc	Beta-carotene: 0.3mg
Fat: 15g	Vitamin C: 33mg
Fibre: 6g	Vitamin E: 0.2mg

Pre-heat the oven to gas mark 6 (200°C, 400°F).

Place the chicken in a roasting tray. Brush with the olive oil and sprinkle with herbs and freshly ground black pepper. Roast in the oven for 20 minutes per lb plus 10–20 minutes extra. Baste the chicken from time to time. To test if it's cooked insert a skewer into the thickest part of the thigh. The juices should run clear. Allow the chicken to stand in a warm place for 10 minutes before carving.

Low-Fat Gravy

Makes 300ml (½pt)

Traditional gravy contains a high level of saturated fat as it is made with meat juices. This recipe is a tasty low-fat alternative that can be used for all meat dishes. Miso is a savoury paste made with fermented rice, barley or soya beans. Different types of miso are available from health food shops. White miso has a mild flavour, while brown miso makes a rich, dark gravy. Miso contains salt, so there is no need to add any more to season the gravy.

450ml (¾pt) chicken stock
1 tbsp miso
juice of 1 orange
black pepper

PER SERVING:	
Kcals: 21Kc	Beta-carotene: Trace
Fat: 0.6g	Vitamin C: 4.7mg
Fibre: 0.2g	Vitamin E: Trace

Warm the chicken stock in a saucepan. Mix together the miso paste with the orange juice and stir into the chicken stock. Season with freshly ground black pepper. Bring to the boil, reduce the heat and simmer for 15–20 minutes until the liquid has reduced in volume by one third. Serve hot. Any remaining gravy can be used as the basis for chicken or mixed vegetable soup.

Apricot Stuffing

To stuff one 1.75kg (4lb) chicken. (Serves about 5.)

175g (6oz) dried apricots, chopped
175g (6oz) fresh, wholewheat breadcrumbs
½ tsp cold-pressed olive oil
freshly ground black pepper

PER SERVING:	
Kcals: 209Kc	Beta-carotene: 0.3mg
Fat: 1g	Vitamin C: 1mg
Fibre: 6g	Vitamin E: 0.1mg

Soak the chopped apricots in cold water for about 30 minutes or until plump and soft. Stir into the breadcrumbs. Add the lemon juice, olive oil and freshly ground black pepper. Work some of the stuffing firmly over the breast and secure the neck flap to keep the stuffing in place. Spoon the remaining stuffing inside the cavity of the chicken.

Fast Fish Risotto

Serves 2

This risotto is a good way to use up pre-cooked rice, and the frozen peas are an excellent source of fibre and protein. Tinned fish such as tuna or salmon may be substituted for the fresh oily fish.

100g (4oz) fresh oily fish (e.g. mackerel or herring)
1 onion, peeled and finely chopped
1 tbsp cold-pressed olive oil
6 heaped tbsps cooked brown rice
150g (5oz) frozen peas
1 tbsp freshly chopped basil and parsley

PER SERVING:

Kcals: 289Kc	Beta-carotene: 0.3mg
Fat: 10g	Vitamin C: 54mg
Fibre: 5.3g	Vitamin E: 1.9mg

Cook the fish under a hot grill for about 5 minutes, turning it once. Allow to cool slightly, then flake the fish flesh into large pieces. Heat the oil in a large frying pan and lightly fry the onion. Add the fish, the rice and peas. Stir continuously to prevent the mixture sticking to the sides of the frying pan while heating through for about 3 minutes to cook the peas. Garnish with the chopped basil or parsley before serving.

Penne with Clams

Serves 4-6

This is one of my all-time favourites. You can use tinned clams packed in brine or fresh ones still in their shells. Use either fresh Tomato Sauce or one of the ready-made tomato sauces that can be bought in jars. Mussels may also be used instead of clams.

1 tbsp olive oil
4 cloves garlic, crushed and chopped
50g (2oz) onions, finely chopped
200g (8oz) fresh tomato sauce (see page 174)
450g (1lb) pasta shells or spinach fettucine
1.5kg (3lbs) fresh clams, well scrubbed or 350g (12oz) tinned clams
salt and black pepper
freshly chopped parsley

PER SERVING:	
Kcals: 372Kc	Beta-carotene: 2.8mg
Fat: 2.4g	Vitamin C: 23.5mg
Fibre: 3.8g	Vitamin E: 0.4mg

Heat the oil in a large frying pan, add the garlic and onions and stir until softened. Add the tomato sauce and simmer for 5 minutes. Meanwhile, cook the pasta until al dente (slightly firm). Steam open the clams by cooking in a steamer above a pan of boiling water. The clams are cooked when all the shells have opened (do not overcook or they will become tough). Remove the clams and add to the tomato sauce, complete with shells. If using tinned clams add them to the sauce at this stage. Season with salt and pepper. Place the pasta in a large serving dish and top with the clam sauce. Sprinkle with chopped parsley and serve immediately.

Asparagus and Mushroom Risotto

Serves 2 as a main dish, or 4 as a starter

To make this tasty light supper dish even more exotic add a pinch of saffron to the cooking liquid. Also, try mixing two types of rice (e.g. brown basmati and brown Italian rice) for added variety.

100g (4oz) brown rices (mixed if possible), well rinsed
475ml (16fl oz) water
1 large onion, peeled and finely chopped
few strands of saffron (optional)
100g (4oz) fresh asparagus, trimmed
2 tsp cold-pressed olive oil
100g (4oz) mushrooms, finely chopped
2 tbsp chopped fresh parsley
freshly ground black pepper
juice of ½ lemon

PER SERVING:	
Kcals: 310Kc	Beta-carotene: 0.3mg
Fat: 3.5g	Vitamin C: 114mg
Fibre: 7.6g	Vitamin E: 1.7mg

Gently heat a heavy-based saucepan on top of the stove, add the rice and stir with a wooden spatula for 1 minute until lightly toasted. Add the water, onion and saffron, if using. Bring to the boil, cover and simmer for 20 minutes. Meanwhile, chop the asparagus into short lengths, reserving the tips for garnish. After the 20 minutes' cooking time add the lengths of asparagus and simmer for another 10–15 minutes until the rice is soft. In a separate pan, gently heat the olive oil and lightly sauté the asparagus tips. Remove from the pan and drain on kitchen paper. Stir the chopped mushrooms and parsley into the cooked rice mixture. Season with black pepper, stir in the lemon juice and serve garnished with the asparagus tips.

Prawns with Gazpacho Dressing

Serves 4

This dinner party dish is ideal for preparing in advance. The dressing also works well with fish, such as hake and trout or even clams, lobster and crab.

20-24 large prawns, cooked

For the dressing:
¼ cucumber, roughly chopped
1 clove garlic, peeled and crushed
¼ red pepper and ¼ yellow pepper, de-seeded and chopped
1 spring onion, sliced
1 tbsp tomato purée
150ml (¼pt) olive oil
1 tbsp wine or cider vinegar
1 tsp fresh oregano, chopped
salt and ground black pepper

For the garnish:
50g (2oz) watercress
1 lime, cut into quarters

PER SERVING:	
Kcals: 151Kc	Beta-carotene: 12.6mg
Fat: 1.6g	Vitamin C: 195.3mg
Fibre: 5.5g	Vitamin E: 0.1mg

Wash and peel the prawns before arranging on a shallow dish. To make the dressing place the cucumber, garlic, peppers and spring onion in a blender or food processor and whizz until finely chopped. Add the tomato purée, olive oil, vinegar and chopped oregano and process until smooth. Season with salt and pepper before pouring over the prawns. Decorate with watercress and lime wedges.

Spinach with Yogurt Dressing

Serves 4

150ml (¼pt) natural low-fat, live yogurt
1 tbsp olive oil
1 tbsp lemon juice or cider vinegar
1 tsp finely chopped onion
1 tbsp chopped fresh mint
1 clove garlic, peeled and split in two
225g (8oz) fresh, young spinach leaves

For the garnish:
A few sprigs of fresh mint
2 radishes, thinly sliced

PER SERVING:	
Kcals: 45Kc	Beta-carotene: 5.3mg
Fat: 1g	Vitamin C: 37.3mg
Fibre: 1.7g	Vitamin E: 1.8mg

Combine the yogurt, olive oil, lemon juice or cider vinegar, onion and mint to make the dressing. Place the garlic
pieces in the dressing or, for a stronger garlic flavour,
squeeze the juice from the clove into the dressing. Toss
the spinach leaves in the dressing and chill for one hour.
Garnish with the mint leaves and radish slices before
serving.

Healthy Hash Browns

Serves 4

This is a low-fat version of America's favourite fried potato dish. Always use organically grown potatoes when possible as they are not sprayed with anti-sprouting chemicals which do not wash off.

2 tbsp olive oil
450g (1lb) potatoes, scrubbed
1 medium onion, finely chopped
2 cloves garlic, crushed and chopped
1 tsp cayenne pepper
salt and black pepper
1 tbsp chopped parsley to garnish

PER SERVING:

Kcals: 118Kc	Beta-carotene: Trace
Fat: 0.7g	Vitamin C: 43.4mg
Fibre: 3g	Vitamin E: 0.3mg

Heat the oil in a large frying pan, wiping away any excess with kitchen paper towel. Add the onions and garlic and stir well. Cut the potatoes into thin slices and add to the oil. Press down with the back of a wooden spoon, sprinkle with cayenne, salt and pepper to taste. Cover the pan with a lid and turn down the heat so the potatoes gently cook through. Once they are cooked, turn the heat up to brown them on the outside. Divide the potatoes in half and flip over to brown the other side. Remove from the pan and blot on kitchen paper towel to remove all excess oil before serving.

Chips in Jackets

Serves 4

We all love chips, even though they are so full of fat, and they are especially hard for children to give up. Instead of banning them altogether, try this low-fat recipe which is a much healthier alternative.

1 tbsp olive oil
1 tsp garlic purée or garlic oil
450g (1lb) large potatoes, scrubbed
salt and black pepper

PER SERVING:	
Kcals: 124Kc	Beta-carotene: Trace
Fat: 0.3g	Vitamin C: 14.5mg
Fibre: 2.8g	Vitamin E: 0.2mg

Pre-heat the oven to gas mark 6 (200°C, 400°F).

Mix together the olive oil and garlic. Use a sharp knife to slice the potatoes lengthways in half, then into long segments, like an orange. Place the potato 'chips' on a non-stick baking tray. Brush with the oil and garlic mixture and lightly season with salt and pepper. Bake for 30–40 minutes, or until golden brown.

Frozen Pea Fritters

Makes 10 fritters

These bright green fritters taste delicious and are popular with children. They are full of fibre and vitamins and are also fun to make, so get the kids to help and be sure they eat up their greens. Served with grilled tomatoes or topped with a spoonful of passata (sieved tomatoes).

225g (8oz) frozen peas
1 egg, separated
1 tsp cayenne pepper
100g (4oz) chick pea (gram) flour
pinch of salt

PER FRITTER:	
Kcals: 61Kc	Beta-carotene: 0.2mg
Fat: 1g	Vitamin C: 2.3mg
Fibre: 1.1g	Vitamin E: 0.2mg

Pre-heat the oven to gas mark 3 (160°C, 325°F).

Defrost the frozen peas by piercing a hole in the bag and cooking on medium in the microwave for 1–2 minutes. Alternatively, simmer in boiling water for 3–4 minutes. Remove from the heat and drain. Place the peas, egg yolk and cayenne pepper in a food processor and whizz until the mixture is a thick paste. Beat the egg white until stiff and stir into the mixture. Stir flour into mixture and shallow fry on both sides. Drain on kitchen paper and keep the first batch warm in the oven while you cook the rest.

ACE Tip: Use the minimum amount of oil necessary for frying. Either use a squirt of oil spray on a non-stick pan or wipe a small amount of oil over the bottom of the pan with a paper towel.

Puréed Carrots with Basil

Serves 4

This delicious vegetable dish can be served with fish, meat or casserole dishes. It is worth using extra virgin olive oil as the flavour comes across very well. Any leftover purée can be added to soups, stocks or risotto dishes. It also makes a great gourmet baby food!

450g (1lb) carrots, scrubbed and sliced
2 tsp extra virgin olive oil
2 tbsp freshly squeezed orange juice
1 tbsp fresh basil, chopped

PER SERVING:	
Kcals: 54Kc	Beta-carotene: 19mg
Fat: 0.4g	Vitamin C: 15mg
Fibre: 2.9g	Vitamin E: 0.6mg

Cook the carrots by placing in boiling water. Reserve the cooking liquid for future use as a vegetable stock or soup base. Place the cooked carrots in a food processor or liquidizer. Purée until smoooth. Add the olive oil, orange juice and chopped basil. Purée again and serve immediately while still hot.

Red Cabbage with Apple

Serves 4

This delicious side dish is cooked like a stir-fry, so you need to watch it cooking on top of the stove. Alternatively, it can also be baked in an ovenproof dish for 15 minutes at gas mark 4 (180°C, 350°F). Its ruby red colour brightens a pale plate of cooked grains and it compliments chicken and fish dishes well.

1 tbsp cold-pressed olive oil
225g (8oz) red cabbage, shredded
2 eating apples, cored and grated (preferably unpeeled)
1 tsp clear honey
1 tsp cider vinegar
freshly ground black pepper

PER SERVING:	
Kcals: 74Kc	Beta-carotene: 0.02mg
Fat: 0.6g	Vitamin C: 36mg
Fibre: 2.7g	Vitamin E: 0.7mg

Heat the oil in a large pan and briefly sauté the cabbage before adding the apples. Then add the honey, vinegar and freshly ground black pepper. Cover and cook gently for 5 minutes.

Spiced Apricots

Serves 4

This is a great summer recipe for using up seasonal fruits and can also be used for peaches and nectarines.

8 fresh apricots
8 cloves
120ml (4fl oz) red wine
grated zest of 1 lemon
2 tsp honey
pinch of allspice

PER SERVING:	
Kcals: 73Kc	Beta-carotene: 0.3mg
Fat: 0.6g	Vitamin C: 10.04mg
Fibre: 1.4g	Vitamin E: Trace

Wash the fruit, stick a clove into each one and place in a non-aluminium saucepan. Pour in the wine, lemon zest, honey and allspice. Bring to the boil, reduce the heat, cover with a lid and simmer for 10 minutes or until the fruit has softened. Remove from the pan and serve warm with low-fat frozen yogurt or fromage frais.

Apricot and Apple Jelly

Serves 4

This is a wonderfully bright and fresh jelly. It is also slightly wobbly, so if you want to turn your jelly out from its mould use about ¾pt of mixed juices. A vegetarian version may be made by using an agar gelling agent available from health food shops.

300ml (½pt) apple juice
300ml (½pt) apricot juice
1 sachet or 3 tsp powdered gelatine
1 passion fruit, pulped (optional)

PER SERVING:

Kcals: 92Kc	Beta-carotene: 0.9mg
Fat: 0.2g	Vitamin C: 3.5mg
Fibre: 1.2g	Vitamin E: Nil

Mix the apple and apricot juices together. Put about one third of the mixture into a bowl. Evenly sprinkle in the gelatine and gently heat over a pan of hot water until all the gelatine has dissolved. Slowly add the remaining fruit juice while stirring, (do not add the gelatine mixture to the fruit juice). Cover and chill until set. Serve decorated with the pulped passion fruit.

Strawberry Sorbet

Serves 4

This recipe can be easily adapted for use with other soft fruits, such as raspberries or blueberries.

450g (1lb) fresh strawberries
2 tsp clear honey (optional)
juice of 1 large orange

PER SERVING:	
Kcals: 51Kc	Beta-carotene: Trace
Fat: 0.4g	Vitamin C: 72mg
Fibre: 2.2g	Vitamin E: 0.3mg

Blend the ingredients together in a food processor until smooth. Pour into a bowl or container and place in the freezing compartment of the fridge (or in the freezer) for an hour.

Remove and allow the mixture to thaw a little, if necessary, then beat well with a metal spoon to break up any ice crystals and return the sorbet to the freezer for at least 5 hours. Allow to soften to room temperature for half an hour before serving.

Prune Clafouti

Serves 6–8

*This deliciously sweet pudding recipe looks and tastes like a cross between crème caramel and crème brulée but it is **much** lower in fat and calories. It is especially popular with children and the quantities given here will make a large dishful.*

½ tsp sunflower oil
100g (4oz) brown sugar
300g (11oz) pitted prunes
2 eggs
1 tsp natural vanilla extract
40g (1½oz) wholewheat flour
250ml (8fl oz) skimmed milk
275ml (9fl oz) low-fat fromage frais

PER SERVING:	
Kcals: 237Kc	Beta-carotene: Trace
Fat: 2.7g	Vitamin C: 2.1mg
Fibre: 3g	Vitamin E: 0.2mg

Pre-heat the oven to gas mark 5 (190°C, 375°F).

Lightly oil a 23cm (or 9-in) ceramic or glass pie dish. Sprinkle 2 tbsp of the sugar inside the dish and tilt to coat the surfaces. Scatter the prunes on top. In a blender, combine the eggs, natural vanilla extract and remaining sugar. Blend until smooth. Add the flour and briefly mix. Add the milk and fromage frais and blend until smooth. Pour the mixture into the dish and bake for about 45 minutes until puffed and browned.

Walnut Apple Crisp

Serves 6

This recipe is a tasty way of using up leftover apples. Walnuts are the best nuts to use, but you could substitute almonds or hazelnuts if preferred. Serve the dish warm with a generous dollop of plain low-fat yogurt or fromage frais.

550g (1¼lb) thinly sliced eating apples
50ml (2fl oz) water
2 tbsp lemon juice
100g (4oz) dark brown or muscovado sugar
50g (2oz) wholewheat flour
1 tsp cinnamon or mixed spice
50ml (2fl oz) olive oil or walnut oil
75g (3oz) coarsely chopped walnuts
25g (1oz) rolled oats

PER SERVING:	
Kcals: 246Kc	Beta-carotene: Trace
Fat: 8g (monounsaturated)	Vitamin C: 9mg
Fibre: 3.5g	Vitamin E: 1mg

Heat oven to gas mark 4 (180°C, 350°F).

In a large, shallow baking dish, mix the apples with the water and lemon juice. In a large bowl, combine the brown sugar, flour and cinnamon and mix well. Stir in the oil until the mixture resembles coarse breadcrumbs. Add the walnuts and oats and mix well. Sprinkle the topping evenly over the apples. Bake for 40-45 minutes or until lightly browned.

Lemon Meringue

Serves 4

This dish is a weight-loss version of the classical lemon meringue pie. It is served without the 'pie' – but with all the taste!

2 lemons (unwaxed), scrubbed clean
1 lime, scrubbed clean
50g (2oz) butter
75g (3oz) castor sugar
1 egg yolk
275ml (½pt) low-fat fromage frais

For the meringue:
2 egg whites
50g (2oz) castor sugar

PER SERVING:

Kcals: 259Kc	Beta-carotene: 0.08mg
Fat: 11g	Vitamin C: 46.6mg
Fibre: 0.6g	Vitamin E: 0.4mg

Use a potato peeler to remove strips of lemon and lime peel. Set to one side. Grate the remainder of the rind and squeeze the juice from each of the fruits. Put this into a small saucepan together with the butter, sugar and egg yolk. Stir over a low heat until the egg yolks thicken the mixture sufficiently to coat the back of a wooden spoon. Remove from the heat, allow to cool and stir in the fromage frais. Chill in the fridge.

Meanwhile, make the meringues by first heating the oven to its lowest setting e.g. gas mark 1 (140°C, 275°F). Beat the egg whites until stiff before adding half the caster sugar. Continue beating until the egg whites form stiff, glazed peaks. Gently fold in the remaining sugar. Cover a baking sheet with a piece of greaseproof paper or baking parchment and spoon on dollops of egg white, leaving a space between each one. Lightly bake the meringues in the cool oven for about 3 hours. When crisp, peel away from the paper and store in an airtight container.

To serve, pour a little of the lemon mixture into each individual bowl, place a meringue on top and scatter with lemon and lime zest.

Apricot and Orange Fluff

Serves 4

The combination of apricot and orange works very well together. These fruits are also a great source of beta-carotene and vitamin C. Use organically grown oranges if you can find them, as their skins have not been sprayed with pesticides which don't wash off.

225g (8oz) dried apricots, soaked overnight
225g (8oz) low-fat fromage frais
1 large orange
2 egg whites, beaten until stiff

PER SERVING:	
Kcals: 193Kc	Beta-carotene: 1.1mg
Fat: 1.2g	Vitamin C: 19.2mg
Fibre: 5.2g	Vitamin E: 0.08mg

Cook the apricots in a little water over a moderate heat for 15–20 minutes, or until softened. Mash with a fork or purée in a food processor. Allow to cool before mixing the apricots with the low-fat fromage frais and honey to taste. Slice the orange in half, remove the pips and squeeze the juice into the mixture. Grate the orange rind into the mixture, keeping a few strips of orange peel aside for decoration. Fold in the egg whites and spoon into individual serving bowls. Decorate with small strips of orange rind or grated zest.

ACE DRINKS

Party Punch

Serves 8-10

This colourful fruit punch has all the taste with none of the alcohol.

600ml (1pt) red grape juice
1.2ltrs (2pts) non-alcoholic sparkling wine
1.2ltrs (2pts) ginger ale
1 large orange, sliced

PER 2-GLASS SERVING:	
Kcals: 110Kc	Beta-carotene: Trace
Fat: Trace	Vitamin C: 11.7mg
Fibre: 0.5g	Vitamin E: 0.1mg

Mix the drinks together in a large punch bowl. Add the slices of fruit and stir well.

Ginger Beer

Serves 8-10

You can use alcohol-free or low-alcohol lager for this unusual ginger beer recipe.

2.25ltrs (4pts) alcohol-free lager
150ml (½pt) ginger beer
1 tbsp grated ginger root
juice of 2 lemons
lemon slices to garnish

PER ½pt SERVING:

Kcals: 81Kc	Beta-carotene: Trace
Fat: Trace	Vitamin C: 12.4mg
Fibre: 0.1g	Vitamin E: Nil

Mix all the ingredients together. Serve over ice with slices of lemon or lime.

Caribbean Cocktail

Serves 8-10

This colourful cocktail adds a splash of colour to any party – and plenty of vitamins too!

2.25ltrs (4pts) carrot juice
1.2trs (2pts) pineapple juice
juice of 1 lemon
lemon and lime slices to garnish

PER 2-GLASS SERVING:	
Kcals: 186Kc	Beta-carotene: 40mg
Fat: 0.5g	Vitamin C: 44.5mg
Fibre: 6.5g	Vitamin E: Nil

Chill the juices before pouring into small glasses. Stir well and garnish with slices of lemon and lime.

Frozen Strawberry Daiquiri

Serves 4

If you're going to drink alcohol, this is a good way of preserving your vitamin and mineral intake at the same time! Strawberries are a good source of vitamin C and potassium.

250g (9oz) frozen strawberries, partially thawed
1 tbsp orange liqueur
1 tbsp freshly squeezed lime juice
6 ice cubes

PER SERVING:	
Kcals: 33Kc	Beta-carotene: Trace
Fat: 0.07g	Vitamin C: 27mg
Fibre: 1.6g	Vitamin E: 0.25mg

Place the partially thawed strawberries in a blender or food processor. Add the orange liqueur and lime juice and mix well. Add the ice cubes and blend until smooth. Serve in cocktail glasses decorated with a fresh strawberry and slice of lime.

Tropical Smoothie

Serves 2

½ ripe papaya
½ banana
50g (2oz) pineapple chunks
1 cup crushed ice

PER SERVING:	
Kcals: 100Kc	Beta-carotene: 0.5mg
Fat: 0.3g	Vitamin C: 84mg
Fibre: 3g	Vitamin E: 0.6mg

A great source of vitamin C, you make this drink by simply whizzing the ingredients together in a blender or food processor.

Chilled Berry Frappé

Serves 2

¼pt skimmed milk or soya milk
1 ripe banana
8-10 frozen berries, e.g. raspberries or blackberries

PER SERVING:	
Kcals: 111Kc	Beta-carotene: Trace
Fat: 0.8g	Vitamin C: 21mg
Fibre: 3.7g	Vitamin E: 0.3mg

Blend the ingredients together in a liquidizer or food processor. This chilled frappé is a wonderfully refreshing summer cocktail.

Strawberry and Pineapple Shake

Serves 2

A serving of fresh strawberries contains fewer than 100 calories, but lots of vitamin C, fibre and potassium. This shake gets the taste buds tingling and is a great idea for breakfast.

150g (6oz) fresh strawberries
120g (4fl oz) pineapple juice
100g (4oz) plain low-fat, live yogurt

PER SERVING:	
Kcals: 93Kc	Beta-carotene: Trace
Fat: 1g	Vitamin C: 50mg
Fibre: 1.4g	Vitamin E: 0.2mg

Wash and hull the strawberries. Place in a blender or food processor. Pour on the pineapple juice and yogurt. Whizz until smooth. Serve as a drink in tall tumblers, or pour over muesli or granola-style cereal.

Mango and Banana Shake

Serves 2

This simple shake is a delicious way to drink your ACE vitamins.

1 ripe banana, peeled
1 ripe mango (or portion of cantaloupe melon), peeled and pitted
300ml (½pt) skimmed milk

PER SERVING:	
Kcals: 174Kc	Beta-carotene: 2.4mg
Fat: 0.8g	Vitamin C: 35mg
Fibre: 3.4g	Vitamin E: 0.3mg

Mix all the ingredients together in a food processor or blender to create a deliciousy frothy shake.

ACE Plan Food Tables

FRUIT (raw unless otherwise stated)	Fibre g/100g	Sugar g/100g	Total fats g/100g	Beta-carotene mg/100g	Vitamin C mg/100g	Vitamin E mg/100g
Apples (stewed)	2.1	7.9	0.1	0.02	11	0.25
Apples	2	11.8	0.1	0.02	6	0.59
Apricots	2.1	6.7	0.1	0.41	6	No data
Apricots (dried)	2.4	43.3	0.6	0.26	9.5	No data
Avocado	2	1.8	22.2	0.02	4	3.2
Bananas	3.4	16.2	0.3	0.02	11	0.27
Blackberries (stewed)	6.3	5.5	0.2	0.07	10	2.03
Blackcurrants (stewed)	7.4	5.6	Trace	0.08	115	0.78
Cherries	1.7	11.9	0.1	0.03	11	0.13
Dates (dried)	8.7	63.9	0.2	0.03	Trace	No data
Figs (dried)	18.5	52.9	1.6	0.06	1	No data
Gooseberries (stewed)	2.7	2.9	0.2	0.04	11	0.31
Grapes, white	0.9	16.1	0.1	0.02	3	Trace
Grapefruit	0.6	5.3	0.1	0.02	36	0.19

Lemons	4.7	3.2	0.3	0.02	58	No data
Melon – cantaloupe	1	4.2	0.1	1	26	0.1
Melon – honeydew	0.9	5	0.1	0.05	9	0.1
Olives (bottled in brine)	4.4	Trace	11	0.18	0	1.99
Oranges	2	8.5	0.1	0.03	54	0.24
Passion fruit	15.9	6.2	0.4	0.75	23	No data
Peaches	1.4	9.1	0.1	0.06	31	No data
Pears	2.3	10.6	0.1	0.02	6	0.5
Pineapple	1.2	11.6	0.2	0.02	12	0.1
Plums	2.1	9.6	0.1	0.3	4	0.61
Plums (stewed)	2.2	5.2	0.1	0.06	3	0.47
Prunes (stewed)	8.1	20.4	0.2	0.14	Trace	No data
Raisins	6.8	64.4	0.4	0.01	1	No data
Raspberries	7.4	5.6	0.3	0.01	32	0.48
Rhubarb (stewed)	2.4	0.9	0.1	0.03	0.18	5
Strawberries	2.2	6.2	0.1	0.01	77	0.2
Sultanas	7	64.7	0.1	0.01	Trace	0.7

VEGETABLES (boiled unless otherwise stated)	Fibre g/100g	Sugar g/100g	Total fats g/100g	Beta-carotene mg/100g	Vitamin C mg/100g	Vitamin E mg/100g
Asparagus	1.5	1.1	0.8	0.53	10	1.16
Broad beans	4.2	0.6	0.6	0.23	8	0.61
French beans	3.2	0.8	0.1	0.18	7	0.12
Runner beans	3.4	1.3	0.2	0.12	10	0.23
Broccoli	4.1	1.5	0.8	0.48	44	1.1
Brussels sprouts	2.9	1.6	1.3	0.32	60	0.9
White cabbage (raw)	2.7	3.7	0.2	0.04	35	0.2
Carrot (raw)	2.9	5.4	0.2	8.12	6	0.56
Carrot	3.1	4.2	0.4	7.56	2	0.56
Cauliflower (raw)	2.1	1.5	0.9	0.05	43	0.22
Cauliflower	1.8	0.8	0.9	0.06	27	0.11
Celery (raw)	1.8	1.2	0.2	0.05	8	0.2
Celery	2.2	0.7	0.3	0.05	4	0.2
Cucumber (raw)	0.4	1.8	0.1	0.06	2	0.07
Leeks	3.9	4.6	0.7	0.58	7	0.92
Lettuce – average (raw)	1.1	1.7	1.7	0.36	5	0.57
Lettuce – butterhead (raw)	1.2	1	1.2	0.91	7	0.57
Lettuce – iceberg (raw)	0.8	1.9	1.9	0.05	3	0.57

Mange tout	3.1	2.8	0.1	0.67	28	0.37
Marrow	0.6	1.3	0.2	0.11	Trace	3
Mushroom	2.5	0.2	0.6	0	1	0.12
Onion (raw)	1.3	5.2	0.2	0.01	5	0.31
Parsnip	2.5	2.7	1.2	0.03	10	1
Peas	5.2	1.8	0.4	0.25	16	0.21
Peas (frozen)	12	1	0.4	0.41	12	0.18
Green peppers	1.6	2.2	0.5	0.24	69	0.8
Red peppers	1.6	6.7	0.4	3.78	81	0.9
Potatoes	1	0.4	0.1	Trace	6	0.06
Potatoes (baked)	2.5	0.6	0.1	Trace	14	1.22
Spinach (raw)	3	1.5	0.8	3.54	26	1.71
Spinach	6.3	1.2	0.5	3.84	26	1.71
Spring greens	3.8	0.9	0.7	2.27	77	No data
Swedes	2.8	3.7	0.1	0.17	15	Trace
Sweetcorn	4.7	1.7	2.4	0.11	1	0.46
Sweet potatoes	2.2	11.6	0.3	3.96	17	4.39
Tomatoes (raw)	1.5	2.8	0.3	0.64	17	1.22
Tomatoes (tinned)	0.9	2	0.1	0.22	12	1.22
Turnips	2	1.9	0.2	0.02	10	Trace
Watercress	3.3	0.6	1	2.52	62	1.46

PULSES (cooked values)	Fibre g/100g	Sugar g/100g	Total fats g/100g	Beta-carotene mg/100g	Vitamin C mg/100g	Vitamin E mg/100g
Aduki beans	5.5	0.5	0.2	0.01	Trace	No data
Black eye beans	3.5	1.1	0.7	0.01	Trace	0.65
Butter beans	5.1	1.5	0.3	Trace	Trace	0.33
Kidney beans	6.7	1	0.5	Trace	1	0.2
Lentils	3.7	0.8	0.5	0.02	Trace	1.28
Soya beans	6.1	2.1	4.2	0.01	Trace	1.13
Split peas	5.1	0.9	0.3	Trace	0.4	2.27

FISH	Fibre	Sugar	Total fats	Beta-carotene	Vitamin C	Vitamin E
(steamed, unless otherwise stated)	g/100g	g/100g	g/100g	mg/100g	mg/100g	mg/100g
Cod	0	0	0.9	Trace	Trace	0.61
Haddock	0	0	0.8	Trace	Trace	1.2
Halibut	0	0	4	Trace	Trace	1
Herring (grilled)	0	0	13	Trace	Trace	25
Lemon sole	0	0	0.9	Trace	Trace	No data
Mackerel (grilled)	0	0	11.3	Trace	Trace	No data
Plaice	0	0	1.9	Trace	Trace	No data
Salmon	0	0	13	Trace	Trace	No data
Salmon (smoked)	0	0	4.5	Trace	Trace	No data
Trout	0	0	4.5	Trace	Trace	No data
Whiting	0	0	0.9	Trace	Trace	No data
Shellfish						
(boiled, unless specified)						
Cockles	0	Trace	0.3	0.01	Trace	No data
Crab	0	0	5.2	Trace	Trace	No data
Lobster	0	0	3.4	Trace	Trace	1.5
Mussels	0	Trace	2	Trace	Trace	No data
Prawns	0	0	1.8	Trace	Trace	No data
Shrimps	0	0	2.4	Trace	1	No data

N.B. Fish and Seafood contain healthy unsaturated fats

MEAT	Fibre	Sugar	Total fats	Beta-carotene	Vitamin C	Vitamin E
	g/100g	g/100g	g/100g	mg/100g	mg/100g	mg/100g
Beef						
Average rump steak, grilled	0	0	12.1	Trace	0	0.32
Lean rump steak, grilled	0	0	6	Trace	0	0.29
Average mince, stewed	0	0	15.2	Trace	0	0.31
Lean mince, stewed	0	0	6	Trace		
Average sirloin, roast	0	0	21.1	Trace	0	0.34
Lean sirloin, roast	0	0	9.1	Trace	0	0.29
Lamb						
Average chops, grilled	0	0	29	Trace	0	0.12
Lean, chops grilled	0	0	12.3	Trace	0	0.1
Average leg, roast	0	0	17.9	Trace	0	0.11
Lean leg, roast	0	0	8.1	Trace	0	0.1
Average shoulder, roast	0	0	26.3	Trace	0	0.12
Lean shoulder, roast	0	0	11.2	Trace	0	0.1
Average breast, roast	0	0	34.6	Trace	0	0.13
Lean breast, roast	0	0	16.6	Trace	0	0.1

Pork						
Average chops, grilled	0	0	24.2	Trace	0	0.03
Lean chops, grilled	0	0	10.7	Trace	0	0
Average leg, roast	0	0	19.8	Trace	0	0.03
Lean leg, roast	0	0	6.9	Trace	0	0
Ham	0	0	5.1	Trace		
Back bacon, lean rashers fried	0	0	22.3	Trace	0	0.06
Back bacon, lean and fat rashers fried	0	0	40.6	Trace	0	0.18
Back bacon, lean rashers grilled	0	0	18.9	Trace	0	0.04
and fat rashers grilled	0	0	33.8	Trace	0	0.11
Poultry and Game						
Chicken, with skin, roast	0	0	14	Trace	0	No data
Chicken, meat only, roast	0	0	5.4	Trace	0	0.11
Duck, with skin, roast	0	0	29	0	0	0.7
Duck, meat only, roast	0	0	9.7	0	0	0.02
Grouse, meat only, roast	0	0	5.3	No data	0	No data
Partridge, meat only, roast	0	0	7.2	No data	0	No data
Pheasant, meat only, roast	0	0	9.3	No data	0	No data
Turkey, with skin, roast	0	0	6.5	No data	0	No data

Poultry – continued						
Turkey, meat only, roast	0	0	2.7	Trace	0	Trace
Rabbit, stewed	0	0	7.7	Trace	0	No data
Venison, roast	0	0	6.4	0	0	No data
Meat products						
Corned beef	0	0	12.1	Trace	0	0.78
Luncheon meat	0.3	Trace	26.9	Trace	0	0.11
Liver sausage	0.5	0.8	26.9	Trace	Trace	0.1
Frankfurters	0.1	Trace	25	Trace	0	0.25
Salami	0.1	Trace	45.2	Trace	8.6	0.28
Pork sausages, grilled	0.7	1.8	24.6	Trace	No data	0.22
Beef sausages	0.7	2.4	18	Trace	23.27	0.22
Beefburgers, fried	1.3	1.4	17.3	Trace	0	0.58
Cornish pastie	1	1.2	20.4	Trace	0	1.3
Pork pie	0.9	0.5	27	Trace	0	0.43
Sausage roll	1.4	1.2	36.2	0.08	0	1.09
Pâté	Trace	0.3	28.9	0.13	6	0.43

OILS	Fibre	Sugar	Total fats	Beta-carotene	Vitamin C	Vitamin E
	g/100g	g/100g	g/100g	mg/100g	mg/100g	mg/100g
Corn oil	0	0	99.9	Trace	0	17.24
Groundnut (peanut) oil	0	0	99.9	Trace	0	15.16
Olive oil	0	0	99.9	No data	0	5.1
Rapeseed oil	0	0	99.9	Trace	0	22.21
Safflower oil	0	0	99.9	Trace	0	40.68
Sesame oil	0	0	99.7	Trace	0	No data
Sunflower oil	0	0	99.9	Trace	0	49.22
Walnut oil	0	0	99.9	0	0	32.11

N.B. Vegetable oils contain healthy unsaturated fats

DAIRY FOOD	Fibre	Sugar	Total fats	Beta-carotene	Vitamin C	Vitamin E
	g/100g	g/100g	g/100g	mg/100g	mg/100g	mg/100g
Milk (whole)	0	4.8	3.8	0.02	1	0.09
Milk (semi-skimmed)	0	5	1.8	0.01	1	0.03
Milk (skimmed)	0	4.8	0.1	Trace	1	Trace
Butter	0	Trace	82	0.43	Trace	2
Cheese (Cheddar)	0	0.1	33.5	0.23	Trace	0.53
Cheese (Brie)	0	Trace	23.2	0.21	Trace	0.84
Cream Cheese	0	Trace	47.4	0.22	Trace	1
Cheese (Edam)	0	Trace	25.4	0.15	Trace	0.48
Cheese (Feta)	0	1.5	18.5	0.03	Trace	0.37
Cottage cheese	0	2.1	4	0.01	Trace	0.08
Cottage cheese – low-fat	0	3.3	1.4	Trace	Trace	0.03
Clotted cream	0	2.3	59.9	0.69	Trace	1.48
Double cream	0	2.7	48.2	0.33	1	1.1
Single cream	0	4.1	21.1	0.13	1	0.4
Yogurt (natural)	0	7.8	3	0.02	1	0.05
Yogurt – low-fat (natural)	0	7.5	0.8	0.01	1	0.01
Eggs (boiled)	0	Trace	10.9	Trace	0	1.11
Eggs (fried – approx fat content depending on type of fat used)	0	Trace	19.5	Trace	0	No data

NUTS AND SEEDS	Fibre	Sugar	Total fats	Beta-carotene	Vitamin C	Vitamin E
(natural)	g/100g	g/100g	g/100g	mg/100g	mg/100g	mg/100g
Almonds	14.3	4.3	53.5	0	0	23.98
Brazil nuts	9	1.7	61.5	0	0	3.3
Cashew nuts	3.2	5.6	50.9	6	0	1.3
Chestnuts	6.8	7	2.7	0	Trace	1.2
Hazelnuts	6.1	4.7	36	0	0	24.98
Coconut	13.6	3.7	36	0	0	0
Peanuts	8.1	3.1	49	0	0	10.09
Pumpkin seeds	10.7	1	45.9	0.04	1.9	No data
Sesame seeds	7.9	0.4	58	0.01	0	2.53
Sunflower seeds	6	1.7	47.5	0.02	0	37.77
Walnuts	5.2	3.2	51.5	0	0	3.83

CEREALS, CAKES & BISCUITS	Fibre	Sugar	Total fats	Beta-carotene	Vitamin C	Vitamin E
	g/100g	g/100g	g/100g	mg/100g	mg/100g	mg/100g
Flour (wholemeal)	9.6	2.3	2	0	0	1.4
Flour (plain, white)	3.4	1.7	1.2	0	0	0.3
Oatmeal	7	1.1	8.7	0	0	1.5
Rice (white, cooked)	0.8	1.2	29.6	0	0	Trace
Rice, (brown, cooked)	1.5	0.5	32.1	0	0	0.3
Pasta (white, cooked)	1	0.5	25.2	0	0	Trace
Pasta (wholemeal, cooked)	3.4	1.3	25	0	0	Trace
Bread (white)	2.7	1.8	47.9	0	0	Trace
Bread (brown)	5.1	1.8	42.9	0	0	Trace
Bread (wholemeal)	8.5	2.1	39.7	0	0	0.2

Biscuits						
Cream crackers	3	Trace	16.3	0	0	1.3
Crispbread (average)	11.7	3.2	2.1	0	0	0.5
Digestive (plain)	5.5	16.4	20.5	0	0	No data
Digestive chocolate)	3.5	28.5	24.1	Trace	0	1.1
Ginger nuts	2	35.8	15.2	No data	0	1.5
Shortbread	2.1	17.2	26	0.13	0	0.8
Cakes						
Victoria jam sponge	1.2	47.7	26.5	No data	0	Trace
Chocolate éclairs	1.1	26.3	24	Trace	Trace	1.25
Fruit cake (plain)	2.8	43.1	12.9	No data	0	1.43
Gingerbread	1.3	31.8	12.6	trace	0	1.5
Doughnuts	2.5	15	15.8	0.01	0	Trace
Mince pies	2.9	31	20.7	0.08	0	0.93
Scones	2.1	6.1	14	0.13	Trace	1.44

N.B. Breakfast cereals – see page 93

JAMS AND CONFECTIONERY	Fibre	Sugar	Total fats	Beta-carotene	Vitamin C	Vitamin E
	g/100g	g/100g	g/100g	mg/100g	mg/100g	mg/100g
Golden syrup	0	79	0	0	0	0
Honey	0	76.4	0	0	0	0
Jam (average)	1	69	0	Trace	10	0
Boiled sweets	0	86.9	Trace	0	0	0
Milk chocolate	Trace	56.5	30.3	0.04	0	0.74
Plain chocolate	No data	59.5	29.2	0.04	0	0.85
Filled chocolates (average)	No data	65.8	18.8	0.04	0	No data
Toffees	0	70.1	17.2	No data	0	No data

GLOSSARY

Antioxidant
A substance that prevents oxidation. Nutrients with anti-oxidant properties include beta-carotene, vitamin C and vitamin E

Ascorbic Acid
Another name for vitamin C

Beta-carotene
A powerful antioxidant, unlike vitamin A which can be made from it. The main sources of beta-carotene in our foods are brightly coloured fruits and vegetables, such as carrots, apricots, spinach and broccoli

Carotenoids
A group of plant pigments ranging in colour from yellow to red. There are over 650 naturally occurring carotenoids many of which have antioxidant properties. However, beta-carotene is one of the most active

Cell membrane
The double layer of fats and proteins that surrounds the living cells of all organisms

Cholesterol
A fatty substance that has many important functions throughout the body. Excess cholesterol may be deposited in the artery lining and lead to heart disease

Degenerative disease
The loss of the capacity of cells, tissues and organs needed for the body to function normally

DNA
The initials stand for Deoxyribonucleic acid, the basic material in the chromosomes of each cell containing the genetic codes of life

Free radical
A reactive particle that contains one or more unpaired electrons, causing it to be highly unstable and sometimes destructive within the body. Free radicals are encouraged by exposure to pollutants such as cigarette smoke. They age cells by damaging their structure and DNA

Lipid
The technical name for any kind of fat or any other fatty substance

Oxidation
The process of using oxygen to release energy from cells. Its side-effect is to produce free radicals

Placebo
A 'dummy' pill given to volunteers taking part in a clinical trial, in which those involved do not know whether they are being given the active substance or a placebo

Polyunsaturates

A fatty acid that contains several double bonds between carbon atoms in its chain

PUFA

The nutritional abbreviation for polyunsaturated fatty acid

RDA

Abbreviation for Recommended Daily Allowance, the amount of a few vitamins and minerals 'needed to satisfy the needs of the population', as advised by governments. This amount does not take into account the additional antioxidant role of the ACE vitamins and is therefore lower than many health experts now suggest

Trans-fats

Fatty acids that have hydrogen and carbon atoms in a double bond on the opposite sides of its normal chain

Vitamins

Over a dozen essential nutrients that the body cannot make from other substances and which must therefore be supplied from food in the diet.

Vitamin A

The active component is retinol or retinyl palmitate. However, this does not have an antioxidant property. The version we need to look for is beta-carotene, which the body can transform into vitamin A. Beta-carotene is the antioxidant version of vitamin A.

Vitamin C

Otherwise known as l-ascorbic acid. This water-soluble substance is thought to be the most important antioxidant in cell fluids. Good sources include citrus fruits, tomatoes, cabbage and strawberries.

Vitamin E

Otherwise known as d-alpha tocopherol, which is the natural form, of dl-alpha tocopherol, which is the less effective synthetic version. Vitamin E is fat-soluble and is found in all cellular membranes. The best food sources are vegetable cooking oils and wheatgerm. We probably do not get enough natural vitamin E from our food and may benefit from taking a supplement.

Useful Addresses
Health Education Authority
Hamilton House
Mabledon Place
London
WC1H 9TX
Telephone 071 383 3833

The Food Commission
3rd Floor
5-11 Worship Street
London EC2A 2BH
Telephone 071 628 7774

The Coronary Prevention Group
Plantation House
Suite 5/4
45 Fenchurch Street
London EC3M 3NN
Telephone 071 626 4844

Further Reading
If you would like to learn more about the important action of the ACE antioxidant vitamins, you may like to read *Liz Earle's ACE Plan* (Boxtree, £4.99). This unique guide reveals the secrets of how to live longer and more healthily with help from the ACE vitamins.

Liz Earle's ACE Plan shows us all how to fight the damaging effect of free radicals to enable us to stay youthful and full of energy. Packed with practical advice and the latest nutritional research, together with a fun quiz for the whole family, *Liz Earle's ACE Plan* is available in paperback from all good bookshops.

If you would like to find out more about the ACE super-vitamins, read *Liz Earle's ACE Plan* which is available from all good bookshops.